FERTILITY FACT

How can I increase my chances of getting pregnant?

In recent years, Western medicine has made great strides in increasing fertility, with innovating techniques such as in vitro fertilization (IVF) and assisted reproductive technologies (ART). But even these remarkable and very expensive procedures are not always successful on their own. Recent findings have revealed that a multifaceted approach combining Western medical technologies with traditional Chinese medicine and holistic medicine can produce dramatic increases in fertility.

GET ALL THE INFORMATION YOU NEED WITH . . .

WHAT YOUR DOCTOR MAY NOT *TELL YOU ABOUT*™ *GETTING PREGNANT*

"Dr. Chang is well known for his integrative East-West approach . . . He has now successfully shown how he integrates the best technology at the disposal of reproductive endocrinologists with a holistic approach that optimizes chances for successful pregnancy. This is must reading for all those having difficulty getting pregnant."

—Allan Warshowsky M.D., F.A.C.O.G., A.B.H.M.,
integrative holistic gynecologist

more . . .

"Dr. Chang offers a full panoply of little known facts that can save you from years of unnecessary heartache."

Julia Indichova, author of *Inconceivable* and
The Fertile Female

"This book offers an innovative 'East meets West' approach to infertility, from medical to surgical therapies options, from female to male factor, and from simple to advanced, state-of-the-art infertility treatments."

—Pak H. Chung, M.D., associate professor and attending,
the Center for Reproductive Medicine & Infertility,
Weill Medical College of Cornell University

WHAT YOUR DOCTOR MAY *NOT* TELL YOU ABOUT™
GETTING PREGNANT

Boost Your Fertility with the Best of Traditional and Alternative Therapies

RAYMOND CHANG, M.D.,
Medical Director, Meridian Medical Group,
with
ELENA OUMANO, PH.D.

A Lynn Sonberg Book

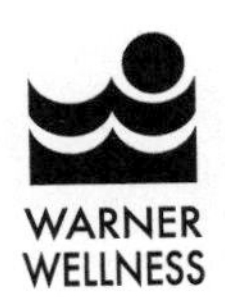

NEW YORK BOSTON

PUBLISHER'S NOTE: The information herein is not intended to replace the services of trained health professionals or be a substitute for medical advice. You are advised to consult with your health care professional with regard to matters relating to your health, and in particular regarding matters that may require diagnosis or medical attention.

Warner Wellness
Warner Books

Hachette Book Group USA
1271 Avenue of the Americas
New York, NY 10020

Warner Wellness is an imprint of Warner Books, Inc.

Printed in the United States of America

First Edition: January 2007
10 9 8 7 6 5 4 3 2 1

Visit our Web site at www.HachetteBookGroupUSA.com

Library of Congress Cataloging-in-Publication Data
Chang, Raymond, 1957–
What your doctor may not tell you about getting pregnant : boost your fertility with the best of traditional and alternative therapies / Raymond Chang, with Elena Oumano.—1st ed.
p. cm.
Includes index.
ISBN-13: 978-0-446-69496-4
ISBN-10: 0-446-69496-7
1. Fertility, Human—Popular works. 2. Infertility—Alternative treatment—Popular works. 3. Human reproductive technology—Popular works. 4. Medicine, Chinese. I. Oumano, Elena. II. Title.
RC889.C43 2006
616.6'92061—dc22 2006007520

To Carolyn, miracle from Erawan,
And her mother, Anne

Acknowledgments

I would like to thank the many who illuminated my path on learning about the miracle of birth and health from the Western as well as the Asian traditions. These individuals include Jeremiah A. Barondess, M.D., and Mary E. Charlson, M.D., who were my mentors during my fellowship training at Cornell/New York Hospital. Thank you also to Woodson Merrell, M.D., in New York for encouragement and support when the Alternative Medicine discipline was still in its infancy, and Dr. Jin Yu of Shanghai, who opened my eyes to the power of acupuncture both in fertility and for reproductive health.

Special thanks need to be extended to Pak Chung, M.D., who has been a true mentor, friend, and colleague from the onset when I became involved in treating infertility over a decade ago, and his colleagues at Cornell's Center for Reproductive Medicine, led by Zev Rosenwaks, M.D., for their openness, confidence, and kind referrals over the years. Special thanks also to James A. Grifo, Ph.D., M.D., for his openness and confidence not only in referring to me but in launching a clinical trial to study the effects of acupuncture on fertility. And I must also thank my Alternative Medicine colleague Pamela Yee, M.D., for her careful review of the manuscript.

Of course, I need to thank Yu Chen, L.Ac., my collaborating acupuncturist for many years, for her many insights and special devotion to fertility and for her special caring kindness to our patients that was indispensable to the success of our program in New York. Special thanks also to my office manager Raquel Acero for taking such special care of our patients and praying for them.

I would also like to thank my highly skilled collaborator, Elena Oumano, who contributed substantially both in form and content to this volume and who was ever patient, versatile, and resourceful throughout the writing process. I am also indebted to Lynn Sonberg, who initially approached me and suggested writing this book. But finally, I must thank my patients, whose persistence and faith taught me to never give up and that there is always a way—or an alternative way—even when conventional medicine has given up—to achieve the baby they prayed for.

Raymond Chang, M.D.

WHAT YOUR DOCTOR MAY *NOT* TELL YOU ABOUT™

GETTING PREGNANT

Contents

Introduction

Why Modern Life Undermines Fertility

For most couples, fertility is not a problem, but for a significant number, the dream of parenthood is elusive. If you haven't been able to conceive, you may feel alone in your predicament, particularly if everyone around you seems to be birthing babies at will. Couples confronted with the issue of infertility are often embarrassed over their inability to conceive and are therefore reluctant to share this with others. That's too bad, because chances are they already know another couple challenged by the same problem. If this is your situation, you've probably been digging up research, seeking opinions, listening to counsel, and, when you still can't get clear-cut answers, are asking, "Why me?"

We have witnessed tremendous advances in conventional medical science's ability to reverse infertility in many couples. Today, even a sixty-two-year-old woman can give birth, with the aid of a donor egg and assisted reproductive technologies

(ART). However, despite the scientific advances of recent years, a key part of the infertility problem is widespread lack of education about reproduction, infertility, and the broad array of fertility-bolstering options that increase odds of conception. For example, some people may not even be clear about the difference between infertility and sterility. *Infertility* refers to a temporary state—the delay of conception or the inability to sustain a pregnancy. *Sterility* describes a permanent state, although even sterility can sometimes be reversed.

If you believe your doctor hasn't told you everything you need to know about fertility, you may be right. First, there's so much to tell. Second, your doctor may not be aware of how traditional Chinese medicine (TCM), which includes acupuncture and other alternative healing options, may successfully treat infertility.

In this book we have gathered together all the information you need in order to make the right reproductive choices. You'll know all your fertility options after we guide you through all the possible causes of infertility—from the obvious to the subtle and often overlooked. You'll find cutting-edge information on the latest fertility-enhancing medical technologies, mind-body discoveries from modern alternative medical research, and ancient fertility-promoting treatments from proven traditional Asian healing modalities.

My vision of medicine and the problem of infertility is, in part, a natural result of living in two worlds. I am originally from Asia, and I came to the United States to attend undergraduate college and medical school. I'm trained in Western medicine, and I also draw inspiration and knowledge from my roots in Asian philosophies and healing traditions, especially TCM. Although my original medical specialty is cancer treatment, working with fertility issues in our clinic has allowed me to create balance in my lifework. Comforting and helping those confronted by death and the process of dying—an all too regrettable accompaniment to a diagnosis of cancer—is countered in my fertility practice by helping bring forth new life.

Let's begin with the hard facts: in a country where 50 to 70 percent of all pregnancies are unplanned, many other couples trying to have children find the road to parenthood quite difficult. Experts estimate that up to 20 percent of North American couples are plagued by infertility, which is sometimes medically defined as not conceiving after one year of unprotected sex. Ten percent of those infertile couples are given the diagnosis of "unexplained infertility." Even under ideal conditions, it's estimated that only 42 percent of a fertile woman's cycles will result in a full-term pregnancy from a fertile partner. Although most experts believe that 90 percent of the time a physical cause is the reason for delayed conception, there can be many possible reasons for not conceiving:

- Sociocultural factors, in particular the widespread pattern of postponing a family until a later age, are a major cause of infertility.
- Common, often asymptomatic, venereal infections can cause scarring in women's reproductive organs and sterility in men.
- High rates of endometriosis, uterine fibroids, and other mechanical problems can prevent a fertilized egg from implanting in the uterine wall.
- Increased emotional and physical stress can turn down the reproductive "thermostat."
- Environmental hazards can cause infertility.
- Overexercise can cause infertility.

- Low body fat and/or poor nutrition can cause infertility.
- Various disruptions within the body's endocrine, nervous, or immune systems can cause infertility.

As you read on, you'll learn the about the following:

- Conventional medical approaches to remedy structural and hormonal blocks to infertility
- TCM and other alternative healing approaches to hormonal obstacles and "unexplained infertility"
- How you can combine conventional medical and TCM for a "best of both worlds" integrative approach to infertility

---

Susan and Ben had shared the dream of parenthood almost from the moment they met, but the "right moment"—when they'd achieved a stable lifestyle with enough time and money to raise a family—didn't arrive until they were in their midthirties. After months of unprotected sex had slipped into a year, Susan and Ben went for a fertility workup. Ben's sperm proved to be fine—millions of little swimmers were ready to impregnate Susan's eggs. The problem was that Susan wasn't releasing any eggs; she wasn't ovulating. Her gynecologist prescribed Clomid, an ovulation-inducing pill that tends to have difficult emotional side effects. Susan endured the emotional roller coaster and the rote sex-on-a-timetable formula: take Clomid, wait seven to ten days, have sex, prop pelvis on pillow, lie quietly for twenty minutes, wait fourteen days for results, and repeat if necessary.

Two expensive in vitro fertilizations (IVFs) didn't work either. Susan and Ben were heartbroken, stranded at the "why us?" end stage of their journey, so when their fertility doctor recommended a visit to our clinic, the Meridian Medical Group, along with one last IVF treatment, they grabbed this "last resort." After only four months of acupuncture, herbs, and simple lifestyle changes, Susan's next IVF treatment took. Nine months later, she and Ben became the proud parents of a beautiful little girl.

It seems as if more and more couples are like Susan and Ben, struggling to be parents and discovering that even the latest, cutting-edge conventional fertility technologies may not be enough.

In cases like Susan's, where the apparent cause of infertility is lack of ovulation, conventional medicine views this as a specific health problem rooted in a specific body part, in particular, the ovaries. In contrast, traditional Chinese medicine views failure to ovulate within a broader context that takes into account the person's entire body and mind (thoughts and emotions) as a fully integrated, interdependent, functioning unit, in which a disruption in healthy function and balance of a single part anywhere in that system can adversely affect the whole. From the perspective of the TCM practitioner, failure to ovulate is not just a problem in the ovaries or even the endocrine (hormone) system. Instead, failure to ovulate is likely to be the end result of another, even more significant and deeply rooted disturbance located elsewhere in the body or mind.

My clinic at the Meridian Medical Group takes this holistic mind-body approach to fertility issues—either using TCM alone or combining TCM and other alternative healing methods when a patient also undertakes reproductive technologies such as IVF. Our program owes a great deal to the work of Dr. Jin Yu, one of the foremost reproductive physicians in China, who pioneered ways to treat infertility with acupuncture, as well as to her scientific studies that confirm how effectively acupuncture treats this medical issue.

Although I met Dr. Yu in New York City, I was able to study her methods in depth during the time I was a visiting professor at Shanghai Medical University in China. I learned about her amazing experiments (which have been published), in which she used acupuncture to induce ovulation in young rabbits that as a species otherwise do not ovulate until they are sexually active. It worked, and the implications are astounding. If we can make otherwise non-ovulating virgin rabbits ovulate with acupuncture, we can biologically readjust nature. Dr. Yu's experiments proved that we can alter an animal's biological functioning despite its natural programming. (And we too are animals.) Patients were queuing up at the front door of Dr. Yu's clinic to be treated. Well known throughout China, Dr. Yu has had amazing success treating women's infertility and menstrual problems with only acupuncture and herbs.

Practitioners of TCM have been using acupuncture and herbs to help women become pregnant for centuries; Dr. Yu was a pioneering TCM practitioner because she applied Western methods of scientific inquiry and rigorous studies to demonstrate clearly that acupuncture and herbs work.

After my studies in China were finished, I invited Dr. Yu to visit our clinic in New York, and together we developed a program to treat infertility with acupuncture and herbs. Our program eventually expanded to include other mind-body modalities, with emphasis on nutrition, stress management, relaxation techniques, visualizations, and hypnosis. Our experience with our patients led me to develop another key component of our fertility treatment—an evolution-based theory of infertility that can make all the difference for you.

As recently as the year 2000, hardly any Western fertility specialists were aware that acupuncture helps increase fertility, yet today it is common knowledge based on our results and publications. Our results have won the confidence of leading doctors at major fertility clinics in New York City and elsewhere in the nation, such as the programs at Cornell and New York University. We have been conducting joint trials with these and other fertility centers, as well as providing complementary care for patients who are also undergoing in vitro fertilization treatments at the centers. In addition, we treat patients who seek out our services for TCM and alternative treatment only—acupuncture along with the individualized mind-body programs we develop for each individual, according to his or her needs.

Most of our patients, though, are referred by fertility centers, many after several unsuccessful attempts with IVF. In our experience, with acupuncture and other holistic strategies we can easily improve the success rate of IVF by up to 30 or 40 percent. Our high success rate also provides hope to those who have been deemed ineligible for conventional fertility programs because of poor ovarian reserve (lack of sufficient viable eggs), even in very resistant cases.

Most of what we have learned in our clinic and what we practice is in this book, so it can be your step-by-step resource for overcoming infertility. In it, you will learn about all the possible causes of infertility. You will be guided through a diverse range of fertility-boosting strategies culled from modern medical science, traditional Asian healing wisdom, and new alternative and holistic approaches so you can make the right choices. You'll know when surgery might be necessary. You'll also understand why TCM can be the most effective "natural" system to help you conceive and deliver a healthy child, one you can use alone or in combination with the any of the modern conventional fertility-enhancing procedures grouped together as assisted reproductive technologies (ART). With the information you'll gather here, you'll know what to do and what not to do in order to optimize your chances for conceiving and bearing a healthy child. You may be surprised to learn that many of our fertility strategies are no more than painless, health-promoting adjustments to your overall lifestyle.

You may be even more surprised to learn how profoundly your mind can impact your ability to conceive and bear a child. You'll learn how the deepest part of the human mind, which we refer to as innate wisdom or collective unconscious, can affect your ability to reproduce. In fact, as your read further, you will understand why overcoming infertility can be a matter of understanding and harnessing your built-in survival instinct to improve your odds of reproduction.

Some information you'll read here overturns long-held but mistaken "rules" of conception; but if you allow it, this book can guide you to preparing your mind and body for the gift of a child.

Chapter 1

A Complementary View of Fertility: The Turns of Fortune's Wheel

As you're reading, you may be planning ahead for a future pregnancy or you may be in the midst of intense hormonal treatments. You may have tried IVF without success. Or you may not be seeking medical treatment at all, simply growing increasingly frustrated over the number of months you've been trying to achieve a successful pregnancy. You may believe it's your fault, yet statistics indicate the cause of infertility is almost as likely to rest with your partner as with you.

Approximately 35 percent of fertility problems are caused by the man's issues, another 35 percent are caused by tubal and pelvic problems in the woman, 15 percent from ovulation dysfunction, 5 percent by immunological, anatomic, or thyroid problems, and 10 percent are attributed to "unknown" causes.

It is important to keep in mind that while studies indicate that one in ten women between the ages of fifteen and forty-four years old will experience infertility, more than 95 percent of couples who seek treatment will not need to undergo advanced reproductive techniques such as in vitro fertilization in order to conceive. Of the 10 percent of infertile couples diagnosed with "unexplained fertility," almost half will conceive within three years. As a general rule, of couples trying to conceive:

- 57 percent succeed within three months
- 72 percent succeed within six months
- 80 to 85 percent succeed within one year
- 90 percent succeed within two years

HOW CONCEPTION OCCURS

Before we explore what can go wrong, let's go through what happens when everything works. The fertilization process takes approximately twenty-four hours, and it begins with ejaculation. Immediately after being deposited in the vagina, semen coagulates—perhaps as a defense mechanism against the vagina's acidic environment, which allows only about 10 percent of sperm to survive the first ten minutes inside. After about twenty minutes, the sperm become fluid again and swim up to the cervix, where protein strands in cervical mucus that are present only just before or during ovulation carry the sperm into the uterus. Since the released egg is viable for twelve to twenty-four hours and sperm live for forty-eight to seventy-two hours, the window of opportunity opens for only about two to three days. Some experts believe that the chance for conception increases if the woman and man experience orgasm simultaneously, because the rhythmic contractions of vagina and uterus during orgasm help propel the sperm closer to the cervix. On the other hand, if the woman experiences orgasm before the man ejaculates, that could lessen chances for conception.

Among the hundreds of sperm that reach the uterus and then the fallopian tubes, some become lost or embedded in the lining of the fallopian tubes. By this point, the heads of the sperm have lost their protective coating, so they can penetrate the egg. (During "sperm washing," a procedure used in artificial or assisted conception, this protective membrane is removed artificially.)

Once a sperm reaches and penetrates the egg, the egg undergoes biochemical changes to ensure no other sperm can enter it, and the sperm and egg combine their genetic material. Unlike egg follicles that retire gracefully once a victorious follicle declares itself the "follicle of the month"—the one with the egg that can be fertilized to create new life—sperm rushing out the testes upon ejaculation compete furiously to beat each other to the finish line. They even refuse to accept defeat after one sperm has penetrated the egg and the winner has been declared, by continuing their attempts to enter the egg.

The fertilized egg then takes a four-day journey to the uterus, where it secretes a hormone called human chorionic gonadotropin (HCG) (detectable by home pregnancy kits) and implants itself in the uterine lining. If the egg doesn't make it to the uterus, it can grow in the fallopian tube, forming what is known as an ectopic, or tubal, pregnancy that must be removed surgically. This is more common in women with scarring from endometriosis, sexually transmitted diseases, or previous pelvic surgery.

Structural problems that can cause ectopic pregnancy or infertility also include fibroids and other malformations. All reproductive specialists—conventional, alternative, and TCM—agree on at least a single point: that "mechanical" or structural reproductive obstacles to fertility must be treated before any other problems are addressed and a successful pregnancy can occur.

WHAT IS INFERTILITY?

For a couple, infertility is defined as being unable to become pregnant after one year of steady, unprotected intercourse. Infertility is the *reduced* ability to have a child. Infertility is not sterility, that is, a lifetime verdict that means you will never have a child. Infertility leaves open the possibility that you *can* have a child at some point. In the up to 20 percent of all couples who are infertile, only 1 to 2 percent of them are actually sterile.

For most couples, infertility is a temporary crisis, one that can be overcome. Even better news, once you are armed with the information and strategies you'll learn here, your chances of a pregnancy that results in the birth of a healthy child will be even greater.

In general, several possible factors hamper fertility in women:

- Lack of ovulation (release of eggs from the ovary) due to hormonal imbalance or cysts in the ovary
- Failure of tubes to carry eggs from the ovary to the uterus, often due to scarring (adhesions) of the fallopian tubes caused by endometriosis, or infections such as gonorrhea and chlamydia, or prior surgery

- Irregular ovulation accompanied by poor cervical mucus that damages sperm or impedes their progress
- Implantation issues in which the embryo cannot implant itself in the uterine lining, caused by fibroid tumors, endometriosis, adhesions, infection, or prior surgery
- The subtle, energetic mind-body imbalances that conventional medicine rarely diagnoses or treats (We will deal with this often overlooked important cause of infertility in women, especially in chapter 11.)

Common causes of infertility in men include:

- Sexual dysfunction (erectile dysfunction or impotence)
- Low sperm count (too few sperm in the ejaculate fluid)
- Low sperm motility (the sperm are not good swimmers)
- Malformation of the sperm
- Blocked sperm ducts

No single fertility treatment is ever successful for everyone, but research has shown that a combination of simple treatments and precautionary measures can greatly enhance a couple's odds of conceiving. This is where TCM is so helpful, either by itself or in partnership with modern Western medical techniques.

SEEING THE BODY AS A WHOLE

Before we talk about what traditional Chinese medicine and other alternative and complementary approaches can do for you, it's worth understanding what these healing modalities really are. Although these approaches are diverse, they share certain principles:

- First, do no harm. TCM and other alternative health care providers generally begin by prescribing less invasive and risky strategies, such as diet and other lifestyle changes, than conventional physicians prescribe.
- Focus on the person, not the disease. TCM and other alternative and complementary practitioners view mind, body, and even spirit as unified and interactive. Women and men also are viewed as part of the environment, so any element in this integrated whole can play a part in creating illness or dysfunction.
- Activate and rebalance energy. TCM and other alternative healing modalities assume an energy force moves within all humans and throughout the natural world. Proper activation of that energy creates good health, so a doctor's role is to help activate that energy in appropriate ways.
- The body, not the doctor, heals. TCM and other alternative practitioners aim to assist your body to activate its own built-in healing mechanisms.
- Allow time for healing to occur. TCM and other alternative practitioners believe that in order for true healing to occur, the body needs time to rebalance and repair. The healing may proceed slowly, but it will be more dramatic, profound, and lasting.
- Look for causes. TCM and other alternative practitioners are less interested in suppressing uncomfortable symptoms than they are in tracking down and addressing root causes. Otherwise, true healing cannot happen.

We can see that regardless of their different terminologies and strategies, TCM and other forms of alternative or holistic healing are directed toward a common goal: treating the whole person and stimulating the body's own self-healing and balancing abilities so optimum health and fertility are recovered naturally.

In the following chapter, we will lead you through the principles of traditional Chinese medicine and show you how it can boost your fertility, whether you use it alone or in combination with assisted reproductive technologies. For now, let's explore how the approach and philosophy of TCM and other alternative healing modalities differ from those of conventional Western medicine.

In general, conventional Western medicine (including the specialty of fertility) tends to see the body *mechanically*—as a collection of organs, any of which may be problematic and need to be treated or repaired. This is a mechanic's point of view—you repair this part or replace that part. It's as if our bodies were automobiles: if a car is low on gas, you add gas. If it needs a new oil filter, you put in an oil filter. If a part of the engine isn't working right, you fix or replace it.

The increasing interest in holistic approaches is also a reaction to Western medicine's overspecialization in which the body systems are viewed as separate from one another. Within this limited and mechanistic model, doctors and patients cannot understand why if everything has been fixed and all the right switches turned on, it still doesn't work. This is why doctors are so puzzled over "unexplained infertility," the category designated to a significant percentage of women who are apparently fertile and healthy but still unable to become pregnant. If this is your situation, you are probably saying something like this: "I had timed our intercourse to the egg's release, my partner's sperm tested well, so why haven't I conceived?" In this day and age of reason and science, we expect our bodies to be as reliable and predictable as the machines we build to make our lives so much easier, and we demand clear-cut answers when something doesn't work as it should.

In contrast to conventional Western medicine's mechanical and specialized view, traditional Chinese medicine approaches the entirety of the mind-body-spirit complex *functionally*. A *functional* approach, such as how we treat patients who come to our clinic, tailors a comprehensive program to the individual needs of each patient and continually modifies that program in order to address the patient's evolving and changing condition. We are in accord with all fertility experts—conventional or TCM—in first checking for and ruling out all structural impediments to fertility. For example, if surgery is necessary, such as in the case of very large uterine fibroids that prevent conception and implantation of the embryo, it must be done before our TCM treatment can take place. Key to our success is encouraging our patients to adopt the most constructive attitude possible toward the fertility process. Miraculously, even in very difficult cases, where every possible conventional approach has failed, an integrative therapy such as the program we offer often leads to success.

TRADITIONAL CHINESE MEDICINE AND THE WHEEL OF FORTUNE

The foundation of our clinic's holistic approach to infertility is traditional Chinese medicine. When many people think of TCM, they think "acupuncture." Yet TCM is a comprehensive health system that also includes its own special diagnostic methods, specific herbs, diet, exercise, massage, and sometimes meditation and physical disciplines. All these treatments are founded on TCM's underlying philosophical approach to all life issues, including fertility.

One principle of the TCM philosophy is that the same energies responsible for creating and governing the universe are also present within the human body, where they control your health and fertility. Studying the body, then, is a way to explore the nature of the universe.

A second principle of TCM is one we in the West often fail to appreciate, the karmic influence of fortune, the fact that our lives are not meant to be entirely under our control. We are, after all, subject to the vicissitudes of chance. The notion of fortune or the wheel of fortune is common to many world cultures, not only traditional Asian societies. In fact, the word *fortune* is associated with Fortuna, a Roman goddess of fertility. The principle of fortune as it relates to fertility becomes clear if you ask yourself the following question: Who gave me an ironclad guarantee that if everything is "normal," I am guaranteed pregnancy and a healthy child?

Do not be discouraged by the element of fortune, as your chances can be improved by our holistic approach. You'll discover that taking fortune into account can actually increase your chances of parenthood.

ZEN AND THE ART OF FERTILITY

A modern spiritual classic first published in 1953 by Eugen Herrigel called *Zen in the Art of Archery* counsels that when it comes to hitting a target—or reaching any goal—aim but never push the arrow. This is equally true when it comes to fertility. We can practice and aim, that is, prepare ourselves in every possible way, but we always must be aware that there are no guarantees, so there's no point in "pushing," especially when the moment comes to pursue the goal. To receive a child means being receptive (remember, the uterus is a receptacle). Receptivity implies passivity, meaning you should not contrive overly in order to receive.

I call this attitude "Zen and the Art of Fertility." Zen philosophy teaches us that sometimes the more we aim and focus, the more often we will be off the mark. A recent study conducted in a San Diego fertility clinic and published in the April 2004 issue of *Fertility and Sterility* found the harder a woman tries to get pregnant—the more focused and worried she is—the less successful her efforts will be. The research team studied 150 women seeking in vitro fertilization or another procedure called gamete intrafallopian transfer (GIFT). The women filled out questionnaires about concerns relating to treatment side effects, surgery, anesthesia, pain recovery, finances, missed work, and having a baby. When the subjects underwent their assisted reproductive technology treatments, those women who worried most about the procedure had 20 percent fewer eggs retrieved and 19 percent fewer eggs fertilized than the women who were less inclined to worry about it. The study actually concluded that the women most worried about conceiving were the least likely to conceive and deliver a baby. On the other hand, those women who took the process in stride and simply allowed it to happen were more likely to become pregnant and have a child.

So, cultivating the philosophy of accepting karmic fortune—as in "Zen and the Art of Fertility"—can increase your chances of getting pregnant. Adopt a positive, healthy attitude in which you "Do your best and let God (or nature) do the rest." In fact, when it comes to parenthood in general, much may be beyond us, despite all our scientific breakthroughs and miracles. Yes, you can optimize your chances by creating the best environment for conception to occur. Once you've rid yourself of the need for certainty—"This has to work!"—you've moved from a state of desperation to a healthier mindset in which you are more empowered, as well as receptive and open to the possibility of new life forming within you.

Chapter 11 tells you exactly how to make this mental-emotional transition. For now, it's enough to recognize that you can help create your own good fortune by recognizing and accepting that conception and childbirth are ultimately acts of nature and can be a matter of luck.

Again, many couples who come to our clinic want to use TCM only, but approximately 40 percent of our patients combine TCM with conventional ART, such as IVF, which has helped many couples. But let's face it, it is an artificial process and it tends to direct women away from their natural reproductive process. In fact, modern medicine in general—for example, medications for menstrual-related discomforts such as premenstrual syndrome (PMS) and various methods of birth control—has distanced women from their bodies, in particular from an innate awareness of the ebb and flow of the menstrual cycle that is so connected to reproduction.

IVF, in particular, is a highly controlled process that involves manipulation of the reproductive cycle and requires adherence to strict timetables, including when to have sex and so on. For example, if you take blood at eight o'clock in the morning and find you're ovulating, you must be ready by ten o'clock for the fertility doctor to transfer eggs from the ovaries.

I counsel couples in my practice not to be too goal oriented or they will stray further from the natural reproductive process, and that is counterproductive. I advise them to do their best to follow all their doctors' recommendations and to integrate the fertility process into their lives as naturally as possible. Afterward, they should try to forget about it, especially if they're undergoing IVF at the same time they're being treated with traditional Chinese medical techniques.

We are sometimes asked "When should I have sex?" The answer always should be "Whenever you both want," because sex should be spontaneous—that's how nature meant it to be. This is a "Zen and the Art of Fertility" attitude that helps you recover a sense of your body's innate rhythms and become pregnant. In fact, this relaxed approach can even increase blood flow to the pelvis, because tension and misery actually tighten the body and restrict blood flow. Restricted pelvic blood flow impedes fertility, as you will learn in the next chapter on TCM. Within the Chinese philosophy of life, health, happiness, and reproduction—all of life—is related to flow—the free flow of energy, of blood, and of all life-giving elements. Nothing can flow freely if you're overly anxious and "uptight."

Zena had been married to Roberto for three years, but by the time they came to us in 2001, they hadn't had any success in starting their family. They were both busy professionals and forty-two-year-old Zena had been based on the West Coast, where she worked as an advertising executive, while Roberto worked on Wall Street in New York City for a full year following their marriage. During that time, they took turns commuting each weekend to be together until Zena was able to transfer to New York in the fall of 1999. However, their schedules remained as hectic as ever. They spent six months looking for an apartment and then moving. Zena was adjusting to her new position in the company while life on Wall Street for Roberto remained frenzied. Both of them were eager to have a child, and because of their age, they started doing IVF in the summer of 2000. After three cycles that yielded no results, they were very frustrated.

They came to our clinic, and I still remember how I could actually feel the stress and frenetic pace of their lives as I listened to their story. My first piece of advice to this couple was to lie back, take a deep breath, and try to relax. When we started Zena on acupuncture, she would doze off during every session because she was so exhausted from lack of sleep and from worry. In fact, she told us it almost felt that the acupuncture sessions were the only times she could relax fully. We referred Zena to our therapist, who taught her visualization and other relaxation techniques you will learn in chapter 11. Gradually, Zena came to recognize that certain material aspects of her life such as her job, her position, her salary, and her advancement should not take priority in her life. Despite the fact that she and Roberto badly wanted a child, with therapy Zena also learned how to give up control and become receptive to a "whatever will be will be" attitude or the mantra you hear repeated over and over in our clinic, "Do your best and God will do the rest." After six months of therapy, the quality of Zena's life changed from tense, hurried, and hectic to evenly paced and composed. Even her relationship with Roberto improved, as did her general health because she was eating better, sleeping more, practicing yoga and visualizations, as well as getting regular acupuncture at our clinic. We also encouraged Zena to indulge herself with manicures, pedicures, and facials and whatever other pampering she enjoyed, especially if they relaxed her. By that time, she and Roberto had settled in their apartment, and Zena had become fond of New York. Roberto reported that Zena had not only mellowed out, but their sex life had improved. In the fall of 2001, they had decided to take a Caribbean vacation. Around Thanksgiving, Zena called the clinic, ecstatic. She was pregnant, apparently without even trying!

When you practice "Zen and the Art of Fertility," you are not only more likely to become pregnant, you also will be better able to accept any outcome. You'll be freer to let go of expectations and move on to explore other options, such as adoption, if you do not wind up with a successful pregnancy. Let's compare fertility to a lottery: you don't buy a lottery ticket with the expectation that you'll definitely win. If you do happen to win, you are happy because you've received an unexpected gift—which is the same attitude you need to cultivate toward fertility. Optimize every possible factor for conception and a full-time pregnancy. Then, step back, be receptive, and allow nature to take its course.

We also can compare the fertility process to applying to college. An applicant puts together the best possible application package—optimal grades and test scores, extracurricular activities, glowing recommendation letters—and tries to have an excellent interview. The applicant with the best chances has not only good test scores and a superior grade point average, but also proof that he or she is a well-rounded person. The first prerequisite is the basics—the test scores and grades. Those basics can be compared to making sure you are cleared for any potential medical fertility issues. If there are problems, you take care of these basics. For example, if there's a large fibroid in your uterus, no matter how balanced your bodily energy is, your chances of becoming pregnant will be reduced, and so you'll probably undergo a surgical procedure to remove the fibroid. The fertility basics involve making sure "the pipes," "the drains," and other reproductive parts are clean and working so everything can flow normally.

Back to applying to college: Let's say the basics—the scores and grades—are great but the applicant is still not granted admission because subtler factors such as extracurricular activities are weak. This situation is like a fertility workup in which everything—sperm quality and count, hormonal profile, anatomy and physiology—checks out as normal. The basics are fine. The couple is apparently healthy, but there is no pregnancy. This is when functional, or non-physical, factors should be explored, including subtle problems, such as weak energy flow, that can't be revealed through scans or blood tests. It's as if everything is working mechanically, but functionally the energy is dim or slow, or the impulse just isn't there. Subtle elements may not be acknowledged as major issues—like grades and recommendation letters or hormonal and structural issues—but they can make or break the success of the application or the pregnancy.

This is why it's sometimes advisable to integrate conventional medicine with alternative approaches in order to put together the most "well-rounded" application possible and give yourself the best possible chance for success.

THE EVOLUTIONARY VIEW OF CONCEPTION

Now, let's explore how your ties to ever-changing nature and your evolutionary past can impact on your ability to conceive and bear a child.

It is simply not enough to address issues of fertility on the level of hormones or such mechanical obstructions as endometriosis, or even from a view of a person as an integrated mind-body system. We must approach fertility from an even broader, more profound perspective that also takes into account a primal drive that tells you when to reproduce and when not to reproduce in order to ensure the survival of our species.

Fertility and the Drive to Survive

Reproduction is an extremely primitive urge, a built-in evolutionary drive we can trace back even to primordial life forms such as algae and bacteria. It has been going on for billions of years. Reproduction could even serve as the definition of life itself—life is that which seeks to replicate itself in the struggle to survive.

As Peter T. Ellison notes in *On Fertile Ground: A Natural History of Human Reproduction*, we "see in the details of our reproductive physiology the imprint of natural selection and the trace of our evolution."

How does this affect your own ability to conceive and bear a healthy child? The study of ecology and Darwin's theory of the survival of the fittest tell us that the species that survive are best able to adapt to their specific environments. We know human physiology is not fixed, and that our major survival tactic is the ability to adjust our bodies continually in response to changes in the environment.

Over the course of human history, nature has fine-tuned us to reproduce in the most efficient way possible. We know this from observing reproductive patterns. We've reproduced more when food is plentiful enough to nourish expectant mothers and their infants, and reproduced less when nourishment is too scarce to support pregnancy and new life. Likewise, during times of danger, war, or famine, when the human race or individual lives—especially new ones—were in jeopardy, fertility rates dropped—our bodies adapted by protecting the few precious eggs we had through shutting down ovulation. This self-protective system in which innate wisdom guides the ebb and flow of our reproduction patterns as a species has kept us going for hundreds of thousands of years. We know too that when other animal species—our relatives—are under duress, they also experience lower fertility. For example, it is well known that animals in captivity have difficulty reproducing. In fact, they seldom reproduce unless they do so after artificial insemination—which is what we humans are doing with IVF treatments. Yet we fail to recognize that overcrowding in cities, for example, works the same way for humans. The evolutionary force within you senses overcrowding and a need to control population growth. What more effective and natural way to adapt in order to accomplish that survival tactic than by lowering fertility? There's too many of us, so the collective unconscious that lives within us all may decide "We won't make more."

Even on the purely physiological level, reproduction is an exquisitely fine-tuned process that can be thrown off easily. As you will learn in the next chapter, reproduction involves not only the harmonious interplay of the entire endocrine system—a hormonal chain of command that sets off a complex chain of molecular signals on cue—but also the cooperation of two other body systems, the nervous system and the immune system. These three systems—endocrine (or hormone), nervous, and immune—are key to the reproductive process *as well as* to creating the prompts that allow your body to make the continual shifts it needs in order to survive in a changing world.

The Grand Plan

Most endocrinologists and other conventional medical reproductive specialists fail to appreciate the grand plan of human reproduction and survival because their focus is narrowed on a biological model of the human, on the reproductive glands and hormones. Even medical experts who take into account the relationship between mind and body rarely explore how infertility rates and *your* fertility issues could fit into this broader evolutionary picture. They do not consider how the deepest part of the human mind that we refer to as innate wisdom or the collective unconscious may impact not only on our physical beings, but also on our individual abilities to reproduce.

Yet even modern-day science knows that we are all connected through a deep level of human consciousness. We know, for example, that the forebrain and cortex—the parts of the brain associated with conscious thought—function independently of the deepest level of consciousness that ties all human beings together.

Traditional Chinese medicine, however, considers many possible factors—from the obvious and mechanical to the subtle and hidden—as influences on your ability to reproduce. It understands that the challenge of infertility requires not only restoring balance within yourself and between you and your partner, but also recognizing how your deep evolutionary programming, which has been in place ever since the first humans walked the earth, may not be in synchrony with your conscious, personal wishes.

Daily Stress and Your "Fertilistat"

If there were such a thing as a thermostat controlling reproduction—a "fertilistat," if you will—then stressful or threatening environments would cue your "fertilistat" downward in order to help you adjust to your environment and optimize survival of the race. So let's take a look at how the stresses of your daily life can interact with the primeval and collective evolutionary drive that dictates how, when, and if you reproduce.

War may not be at your doorstep, but you can witness its sounds and sights every night on your television screen. Your refrigerator may be full of food, but you may be monitoring your diet to make sure you stay fashionably slim. Or you may live in a city that signals to your reproductive "fertilistat" that your environment is overcrowded.

Your deepest consciousness is literal—whether the war is conducted right before your eyes or you take in its images from a TV screen, your deepest consciousness interprets this information to mean you are living in a time of unprecedented *perceived* danger, stress, and anxiety. This *perception* of danger, stress, and anxiety can override even your deepest desire to conceive and bear a child.

So you, the individual, may think this is a great time for you to reproduce, but your deepest level of consciousness is taking in information about war, terrorism, danger, starvation, and overcrowding and sensing that, as a race, we should not reproduce more. There won't be enough food, water, security, or enough of anything else we need to survive. Even the stress of exercise—running or jogging, for example—can cue your "fertilistat" to lower, because running evokes a deep and old instinct of how we escape imminent danger.

What can you, the individual, do? I assure my patients that they don't need to relocate to a deserted island. Instead, I advise them on how to outsmart these powerful and intelligent forces that are telling your body this is not a good time for you to reproduce. You will learn these simple tips in chapter 11, so you will be able to assure your mind-body system that the right time for you to have a baby is now.

Chapter 2

How Traditional Chinese Medicine Boosts Fertility

Scholars place the earliest documents demonstrating the use of traditional Chinese medicine at around 250 BC. Some believe that this safe and effective holistic healing system has been in practice for several thousand years. As we tell our office patients, TCM has been fine-tuned over time. Its original engineers left us a blueprint that tells us how it should be done, so we follow it and it works. Today, TCM is used by millions of people around the world to induce balance in the mind-body matrix to promote balance and movement of life-force energy called qi (pronounced "chee"), as well as blood and other fluid circulation. Like conventional medicine, traditional Chinese medicine works by diagnosing and treating illness. Unlike conventional medicine, however, within the traditional Chinese healing point of view, no single part can be understood except in its relation to the whole.

Within TCM philosophy, imbalances that disrupt fertility

can even originate outside a person's actual physical body. For example, prolonged exposure to overly cold or damp weather can impair health and lower fertility.

You probably know about the most well known element of TCM, acupuncture, a procedure in which fine needles are inserted into, and can be manipulated at more than 365 points in, the body. You may not be aware, however, that TCM also includes a complex and venerable system of herbal treatments, nutritional guidelines, special exercises, and massage as well as other lifestyle modifications. The aim of TCM is not only curing specific ailments, but also protecting sound health so that problems can be prevented before they arise. Acupuncture has had great acknowledgment and respect ever since the seventies, when it first made an impact in this country, and has grown tremendously in popularity over the decades. An increasing number of conventional medical doctors are incorporating acupuncture into their practices, and TCM schools are opening up all over the country, both training practitioners in this venerable practice and teaching them how to practice TCM in tandem with conventional medicine. Because the science of Chinese herbs is so complex, some TCM practitioners use acupuncture as their sole treatment modality; however, others incorporate herbal therapy and other TCM elements in their treatments. Licensing boards have been set up in most states to regulate practitioners and protect clients. Of course, the skill of your acupuncturist is one of the factors that determines the successful outcome of your treatments. In addition, there are many different acupuncture techniques and styles. The cost can vary, and some insurance companies cover acupuncture treatments for only a limited array of conditions that often do not include infertility.

Acupuncture, as well as other TCM treatments, improves

ovulation cycles, even in women with ovarian disorders. It also improves the lining of the uterus, thereby making it more likely that an embryo can embed itself and draw the nourishment it needs to thrive. This lining is like soil in a garden; if it is lacking in essential nutrients, the embryo can't attach itself and grow.

At our center, we use TCM and acupuncture alone to treat infertility or in tandem with conventional fertility-enhancing drugs and/or assisted reproductive technologies such as in vitro fertilization. It all depends on the wants and needs of the patient. The great advantage of using acupuncture along with IVF is there's no possibility of chemical interactions, since all we use for treatment are sterile needles. We are even less likely to prescribe herbs for someone undergoing IVF at the same time as acupuncture to make sure there's no interference with the fertility drugs.

Some people who come to our clinic are "first timers," people who are having trouble getting pregnant and want a natural, health-enhancing strategy to boost fertility. Many of our patients, though, are referred to us by conventional reproductive medicine specialists, usually after they have failed one or more attempts at IVF. Before administering another IVF cycle, the fertility doctors recommend adding our TCM treatment to complement their efforts. As we stated earlier, we have found that our treatments can increase the success rate for IVF by up to 30 or 40 percent. That's a dramatic figure when you keep in mind that the patients who come to our clinic are on average thirty-eight years old and have previously failed two IVF cycles. Some may have undergone as many as ten IVF cycles before they come to us. Of course, these patients' chances of becoming pregnant are significantly lower. In general, your chances for success go down as your age and the number of failed IVF cycles goes up. Yet, one out of three of our patients winds up with a successful pregnancy.

Linda was married for eleven years, suffering from unexplained infertility. Before that, Linda had endometriosis and her husband had sperm quality issues. Throughout their marriage they were told that nothing was preventing Linda from becoming pregnant. After seven years of trying, a doctor suggested IVF, which they tried without success. Just before her eleventh wedding anniversary, Linda noticed her menstrual periods were becoming lighter. A fertility specialist took her FSH (follicle-stimulating hormone) levels and told Linda and her husband that the number was high and indicated premature menopause. He suggested using an egg donor. Two IVF specialists then rejected Linda as a patient unless her FSH numbers lowered sufficiently for two consecutive cycles.

Finally, a good friend of Linda's who knew people with a similar diagnosis who had become pregnant with acupuncture from us recommended me to her for treatment.

Much to Linda's surprise, her FSH levels lowered after her first month of acupuncture treatments. In her second month of treatment, Linda decided to try one more IVF cycle while continuing acupuncture with us. In previous IVF cycles, her egg quality was not good. However, after acupuncture, most of her eggs were rated high quality. Linda became pregnant with her first acupuncture-IVF cycle and gave birth to a beautiful daughter.

Again, keep in mind that acupuncture and other elements of TCM (herbs, nutrition, and lifestyle modifications) work as well alone as do fertility drugs when it comes to improving conception and implantation rates. However, depending on your situation, some sort of assisted reproductive procedure may be necessary.

SCIENCE AND TCM

The moving of energy, or qi, by acupuncture in order to produce adjustments in your body's tissues, nerves, and hormones may seem an ethereal, unproven concept, but scientific research conducted over the past few decades backs up claims that acupuncture stimulates the production of hormones and immune system cells and activates the anti-inflammatory response, creating many beneficial effects, including enhanced fertility.

In a report published in the April 2002 issue of *Fertility and Sterility*, German researchers studying 160 women undergoing IVF concluded that adding acupuncture to IVF increased pregnancy rates by approximately 40 percent. Noted Cornell University reproductive endocrinologists, Dr. Zev Rosenwaks and Dr. Pak Chung, and I conducted a review of existing research and found clear links between acupuncture treatment and a change in the levels of the brain hormones involved in conception. This landmark review, published in the December 2002 issue of *Fertility and Sterility*, showed that acupuncture increases production of endorphins, the "feel good" hormones that play a role in regulating menstrual cycles and, therefore, also affect fertility. Our survey of other research results as well suggests that acupuncture accomplishes this neuroendocrine effect. It seems to strengthen cooperation between two key players in the hormonal chain of command—the hypothalamus and pituitary gland—along with the ovaries, thereby helping them produce the right levels of hormones at the right times to enhance egg production and ovulation. Our survey recommended further study of the role of acupuncture in treating infertility through its impact on that particular aspect of the endocrine system—the hypothalamic-pituitary-ovarian axis.

A 1997 clinical observation study in volume 22 of *Acupuncture and Electrotherapy Research* found that electro-acupuncture, in which pulses of low-level electric current flow through the needles, helps regulate the release of certain hormones. This correction of endocrine imbalance can reduce endometriosis, as well as relieve other gynecological conditions, including fibroid conditions, in some cases, even shrink fibroid tumors.

Another important point we discovered is that acupuncture stimulates pelvic blood flow through a relaxation of the blood supply to the ovaries and uterus. Improved blood flow allows the eggs to receive better nutrition and also improves the uterine lining (endometrium), where embryos are "hatched" and develop into babies. Corroborating research published in the Spring/Summer 2000 issue of *Medical Acupuncture*, by Sandra Emmons, M.D., an assistant professor of obstetrics and gynecology at Oregon Health Sciences University, also reports that acupuncture may directly impact the number of egg follicles available for fertilization in women undergoing IVF because acupuncture stimulates blood circulation.

Additional studies have demonstrated the effectiveness of TCM and acupuncture in treating not only infertility, but also a growing list of disorders either treated by acupuncture alone, or in combination with conventional medicine. The World Health Organization and the National Institutes of Health confirm that acupuncture and TCM may be able to treat addictions, strokes, headaches and migraines, menstrual disorders such as cramps, fibromyalgia and chronic fatigue syndrome, osteoarthritis, back pain, sports injuries, carpal tunnel syndrome, asthma, dental pain, side effects from cancer treatment, depression, pregnancy problems, and, of course, infertility. A 2002 survey conducted by National Health Interview Survey puts the number of American adults who have tried acupuncture at approximately 8.2 million. Only a year earlier, the estimated number was 2.1! Additional ongoing research projects are exploring ways in which acupuncture promotes fertility, as well as its other health benefits.

If you have been trying to conceive, it's important for you to be aware of the proven effects of the balancing and revitalizing effects of acupuncture. Acupuncture:

- Reduces stress hormones that interfere with ovulation
- Increases blood flow to the reproductive organs and glands
- Increases levels of the "feel good" hormones known as endorphins
- Stimulates and normalizes hormone production to promote a balanced endocrine system that allows for more efficient ovulation and fertilization
- Improves the quality of eggs released by the ovaries
- Enhances the uterine lining so the embryo can implant itself successfully and receive proper nutrients (avoiding a miscarriage)
- Enhances the quality of cervical mucus
- *Improves pregnancy rates in women undergoing in vitro fertilization*

WHEN TO TRY TRADITIONAL CHINESE MEDICINE

If you are relatively young and time is not yet a concern, you might want to try TCM first. Your practitioner will decide whether or not herbs, nutritional recommendations, and other lifestyle modifications should also be part of your treatment plan. Pregnancy rates for acupuncture treatments without IVF or any other ART treatment equal the results of conventional fertility treatment with an ovulation-stimulating drug such as Clomid alone—a 50 percent chance of pregnancy within three months. ART treatments are often time-consuming and expensive, and, as you will learn in chapter 7, they do not always work. So, if you haven't become pregnant after one year of unprotected sex, acupuncture is a great choice for your "stand-alone" fertility treatment to stimulate egg production if you cannot use fertility medications or if you'd rather not go the conventional medical route. There's nothing to lose. Treatments are cost effective and benefit your general health. If you are in your early or midthirties or younger and have no reason to suspect structural fertility obstacles, a few months of TCM may be enough to help you get pregnant.

Another choice might be to begin with a basic fertility workup that rules out structural problems. This is especially wise if you are over forty and/or have a history of sexually transmitted diseases (STDs), fibroids, or endometriosis, which can cause such problems as scars (adhesions) and structural blockages. However, having fibroids or endometriosis does not mean you can't get pregnant. It all depends on the severity of the condition, and, as you will learn in chapters 8 and 9 on infertility and hormone imbalance, both problems can be treated successfully through a program involving acupuncture, herbs, nutrition, and other lifestyle modifications.

If you are older and time is a concern, however, you might consider combining acupuncture with ART techniques such as fertility drugs and/or IVF. Keep in mind, though, that the only difference between these methods of promoting ovulation is that acupuncture usually stimulates the growth and release of a single egg, while the fertility drugs work by producing multiple eggs. Of course, if you are past a certain age and no longer ovulating, nothing will stimulate production of eggs that are no longer present.

A note about herbs: Like acupuncture, Chinese herbal therapy works to promote circulation of energy and fluids in the body in order to restore balance and function. *However, you should never take any herbs if you may be pregnant, unless on the advice of your doctor, as some herbs can disrupt the pregnancy.* You'll learn more about how herbs can prepare you for pregnancy in chapter 9.

In short, TCM can help just about anyone experiencing nonstructural infertility. The exception is if your fertility problem involves structural obstacles such as blocked fallopian tubes, a large fibroid tumor, extensive damage to the uterine lining, or anatomical defects. In those cases, surgery is the initial and essential step. However, *after* surgery has removed blocks to a successful pregnancy, TCM can then help promote fertility.

THE COMPLETE TCM HEALING ARSENAL

Acupuncture and Chinese herbal therapy, generally considered the most developed and refined in the world, are only two of the many healing modalities included under the TCM umbrella. In order to fully understand TCM healing and how it can help you, let's take a look at its most important concepts.

The Concept of Qi

Tied to the principle of viewing a person within his or her environment, the concept of qi signifies the constant flow of life force. Qi is an invisible energy force that moves through our bodies and the universe, unifying all life. It moves through the body along a series of invisible energetic channels called meridians that unify an entire mind-body complex, including organs, tissues, and substances (blood, phlegm, qi, other fluids, and food), that is not limited to the Western view of anatomy and physiology. The animating universal energy that circulates through, within, and around us, qi is responsible for our growth and development, as well as for maintaining good health. Whenever there are blocks or disruptions anywhere along the meridians, causing "stagnating" or "insufficient" qi, the various organ and gland systems will receive too much or too little qi. Deficiency conditions cause symptoms of decreased function and strength and tend to be less severe than the more acute and stronger symptoms associated with excess or "stagnating" qi. Pain is a typical symptom of "stuck" or "stagnating" qi.

These energetic disruptions cause illness and dysfunction, including the hormonal imbalances and other problems that impair fertility. Simple yoga and Chinese Taoist practices cultivate energy flow in the pelvis, and these exercises benefit the entire body because all the body's energy currents (acupuncture meridians) pass through the pelvic area. If the qi in your pelvic area is blocked or weak, you lose valuable life energy, as well as blood and lymph circulation. Because the pelvic area is the seat of your energy, your entire mind-body complex will suffer, your brain as well as your ability to reproduce.

Most of us experience an abundance of life-force energy only in our youth. Yet we are capable of conserving, even increasing this energy, well into our senior years. The problem is we do not know how to preserve and channel our qi, let alone how to restore and multiply it in order to enhance fertility. Poor diet, overexercise or lack of healthy exercise, stress, alcohol, drugs, smoking, and environment toxins gradually wear us out. We become listless and chronically tired, even depressed, and this does not bode well for our fertility.

The Dichotomy of Yin and Yang

Folded into the concept of qi is the dichotomy of yin and yang. In TCM, yin and yang refer to polar opposites in the universe—like hot and cold, dry and damp, male and female. Every element, function, and feeling of life has its complementary opposite. When they are in balance with each other, the outer world is harmonious and functions smoothly. The same is true of a person; when the elements of qi, blood, and other fluids are circulating freely in the body, the yin and yang are in balance and the mind-body system creates internal harmony. Within this point of view, illness or a dysfunction such as infertility results from an imbalance in yin and yang, which itself may result from interrupted, insufficient qi, or stagnated qi. As a TCM doctor, I see each person as a unified whole, a mini ecosystem, in which an excess or deficiency of cold, heat, wind, dampness, or dryness affects internal balance and can make the person off balance. For example, if you live in a wet climate, you can have excess internal moisture. Another example is what we commonly call "flu," which in TCM can be an excess of heat, accompanied by fever, redness, and swelling, or as an excess of cold, accompanied by chills and weakness.

The point is that all opposing aspects must be in proper balance within you and between you and your environment in order for you to achieve and maintain peak health and fertility.

Yin and yang imbalance can be subtle, even unconscious, and it can be present between two people, let's say between a man and a woman. In such cases, imbalance between the couple's energy even can prevent them from conceiving a child. For example, I recently saw an infertile woman who finally confessed that she wasn't certain that her partner was the man with whom she really wanted to spend her life. The part of her that sensed she did not have harmony and balance with her partner was unconsciously affecting her ability to conceive. Something inside was telling her the situation wasn't right. On the other hand, when yin and yang balance exists within each partner and between the couple, the stage is set for a baby to be conceived. Yin and yang form a partnership. Two years after this woman left her partner, she married the love of her life and, soon after, gave birth to a healthy child without any trouble.

If you are asking yourself why nothing is working, take a moment to consider the subtle dance between the yin and yang within you, and between female and male elements—with you and your partner.

How Acupuncture Works

Acupuncture involves placing tiny sterile needles in various points along a gridlike map of energy channels, meridians, that span the body from head to toe. Not corresponding precisely to the Western view of organ systems, these are the five main organ networks that govern bodily functions:

- Liver—stores and releases blood and circulates qi
- Heart—propels blood and affects mental function
- Spleen—controls digestion
- Lungs—refine qi and establish the body's rhythm
- Kidneys—oversee reproduction and regeneration

The needles may look lethal to a novice, but acupuncture is actually rather painless and promotes a pleasant sensation of well-being as it restores balance throughout the mind-body complex. The needles are usually left in for fifteen to twenty-five minutes to stimulate more than 365 possible points (plus "extra" points used for specific disorders), thereby moving energy from where it is congested to parts where it's deficient. According to your individual condition, we determine which points to penetrate in order to release energy blocks and restore energy flow and vitality. However, the points most often used for enhancing fertility are usually along the kidney (yin) and stomach and colon (yang) in conjunction with nine other main meridians because they improve blood flow and energy to the uterus and provide a calming effect. Length of treatment depends on your condition, but most fertility cases experience results with two treatments per week for anywhere from a few weeks up to several months.

Whether the direct cause of your infertility is "physical"—let's say due to lack of ovulation—or an indirect result of persistent chronic stress or tension, once acupuncture restores energy flow as well as blood and lymph circulation, your body is able to self-correct, rebalance, and perform at optimal levels.

Acupuncture, as well as other parts of TCM, also can effectively improve fertility—sperm quality and motility—in your partner. In general, acupuncture relieves men of stress, often caused by overwork or even performance anxiety. This is usually accomplished by strengthening the kidney meridian that governs reproduction, thereby increasing sperm production and motility. Most men's first choice of treatment for sperm problems, however, is usually herbs or supplements. In cases where sperm is unable to reach the egg due to low motility or ejaculation problems, conventional fertility specialists may recommend in vitro fertilization after a single sperm has been injected into your egg in the laboratory (a procedure called intracytoplasmic sperm injection [ICSI]). This breakthrough medical treatment offers hope to couples when the man has no or very low sperm count or produces few good-quality sperm and the couple does not want to use donor sperm.

TCM DIAGNOSIS TECHNIQUES

A TCM practitioner needs to be well trained and experienced in tongue examination, pulse reading, and other methods of TCM diagnosis. Before any TCM treatment, we thoroughly assess your health through an extensive step-by-step method that can take anywhere up to half an hour. Only then can we draw up a tentative yet comprehensive treatment plan that will continually evolve as your condition changes over the course of treatment. In most cases, the treatment includes acupuncture. In many cases, treatment will also include nutritional and other lifestyle modifications and herbs. Very often, these TCM strategies are all that's needed for a successful pregnancy.

Step 1: "First Impressions." I begin my evaluation of a patient's condition by observing the color and form of her face and body. I take a moment to initially scan the whole person to check if anything is wrong that I can spot immediately. Sometimes it is very subtle, as in an energy that emanates from the person; other times signs of stress or illness such as a pale complexion, a distraught or anxious manner, or poor hygiene can suggest emotional issues.

Most practitioners of TCM are also well versed in the ancient art of "face reading," or physiognomy, as practiced by many traditional healers. According to TCM, each facial feature may correspond to an organ system or network in the body. The feature's size, shape, coloring, and placement are believed to reveal information about a person's health, as well as certain character traits. For example, your cheeks correlate to your lungs, your brows correspond to your liver, and your lips show the status of your digestive organs. The area around your mouth corresponds to your reproductive organs. Redness above the mouth, then, could indicate inflammation in the prostate or ovaries. Face readers also look at lines, scars, and moles, and the difference between the left side of your face (your inner self) and the right side (the self you show the world). In TCM, the boundaries between psychological and physiological are blurred, so your face becomes a map of who you are, physically and emotionally. The most important bodily part that we focus on is the tongue. The tongue can be thought of as an extension of your upper intestines and reveals many of your body's secrets upon examination. Your tongue's coating, shape, and size may differ according to your health, so we examine the tongue for attributes and qualities to learn more about your inner health state.

Step 2: "Listening and Asking." We check our initial impressions through listening to the patient's complaints, and his or her life story, and follow up with specific questioning.

This is where we work together with you on "solving the problem," because your experience of your condition yields important information, which makes you an expert as well. For example, we may ask about your energy level, if you tend to feel hot or cold, if you have pain, and so forth. We will want to know about your digestion and eating habits—what foods you prefer; patterns in thirst, perspiration, saliva, and tears; frequency and characteristics of bowel movements; frequency, color, sensation, and quality of stream in urination; amount, quality, and patterns of sleep. We may ask about any abnormalities in your sight, hearing, taste, sense of touch, or thought and behavior problems. We are also interested in your work and leisure habits, your capacity for work, your activity level, and whether you travel much. We will also want to know about your level of sexual desire and activity, as well as the regularity, length, quality, color, and sensation of your menstrual cycles. We can usually learn a great deal about possible fertility problems by asking you about all these things, as well as about your medical and family history, emotional well-being, and physical environment. Your answers give us a more complete understanding of your condition, and they also help you become more "in tune" with your mind-body complex and increase your sensitivity to subtle shifts in your condition.

Step 3: "Pulse and Palpating." Western medicine considers your pulse from only two angles—the rate and the rhythm. Your pulse is taken by feeling for the radial pulse on the wrist, located just under the thumb. Arteries carry oxygenated blood away from the heart to the tissues of the body; veins carry blood depleted of oxygen from the same tissues back to the heart. The arteries are the vessels with the "pulse," a rhythmic pushing of the blood to the heart, followed by the refilling of the heart chamber. To determine heart rate, you feel the beats at a point such as the radial pulse for ten seconds, then multiply the number of pulses by six. This is the per-minute total. While the pulse rate measures your heart rate, the rhythm of the pulse reveals if the heart rate is regular or irregular. In conventional Western medicine, there's no further pulse examination.

In TCM, however, at least thirty-two different pulse forms can be felt and interpreted. The pulses tell us a lot about the energy and fluid movement and balance throughout your meridian and organ systems. Generally, we start by taking the radial pulse to check overall strength and condition. We then check various sites up and down on the radial pulse that correspond to the upper, middle, and lower sections of your body. These are termed "burners." The "upper burner" includes the heart and lungs, the "middle burner" takes in the midsection of the abdomen, and the "lower burner" includes the lower abdomen. We check the pulses for surface and deep strength, which reflect the state of internal organs.

We confirm information we've gathered so far about which organ system(s) are affected by looking for other signs and symptoms of disharmony on your body. These signs and symptoms are evaluated sometimes by palpating your body to see which areas may be hot, cold, tight, ropy, or flaccid, indicating disturbed flow of qi or blood. Palpation is not unlike a Western physical exam, although it is not nearly as extensive. An area that is warm to the touch, dominated by heat, is often associated with agitation, restlessness, redness, inflammation, and a reactive sensitivity. Applications of cold or cool substances can relieve this condition, if only temporarily. A cold or cool area is usually associated with symptoms such as cramping, contraction, chill, and depressed function. Applications of heat can provide relief. A damp area feels spongy to the touch, and the patient has a sensation of heaviness or being clogged. The symptoms can include diarrhea, fluid leaking from various sites, and vaginal discharge containing mucus. A dry area means fluid is deficient. Symptoms can include agitation and itchiness and are often relieved by hydration or by applying external moisture.

ACUPUNCTURE TREATMENT

Finally, we gather all that we've learned about your condition and which organ networks are affected so we can draw up a comprehensive treatment plan. When we are evaluating a patient who has undergone a conventional medical fertility workup, or is also undergoing an ART procedure, we combine the wealth of diagnostic information we've gathered from our TCM examination with any laboratory or testing reports that we receive from the patient's conventional physician or fertility specialist. This enables us to pinpoint possible obstacles to conception with greater accuracy. In TCM, the diagnostic process is ongoing as we continue to observe how the nature of your problem evolves throughout treatment. So the treatment itself becomes a key part of the ongoing diagnosis. Your changing condition due to treatment requires continual adjustments in how you are needled and in which locations and/or any herbal remedies you might need.

During the first treatment session, acupuncture needling may be limited so we can see how you respond and recheck our diagnostic assessment. This also allows you to become accustomed to the process. As treatment proceeds, we note how you are responding and adapt the treatment accordingly. Your treatment plan now can include any or all of the following:

- nutritional recommendations
- supplement recommendations
- herbal remedies
- relaxation and meditation techniques and other stress-relieving strategies
- yoga, qigong, and other qi-balancing disciplines
- other lifestyle adjustments

What to Expect in a Typical Acupuncture Session

We will take your pulses and ask questions about how you are feeling, and then check your tongue.

You lie down and we insert new and sterile acupuncture needles into prescribed points called "acupoints" along your meridians, your energy channels. You may be afraid the first time you are treated, but after the initial visit, you should be relaxed.

The depth a needle is inserted depends on your symptoms, where the point is located on your body, the amount of your body fat, your size, age, and state of health, as well as the particular acupuncture style your practitioner uses.

We may also stimulate the needles manually every so often, or use a low-voltage electric current and/or infrared heat treatment. Some practitioners follow acupuncture treatment with cupping, in which a vacuum is created in a glass "cup" by lighting a ball of alcohol-soaked cotton, passing it inside the cup, and then placing the cup over acupuncture points. This is used to relieve stagnation, or blood stasis, and stimulate circulation.

We sometimes also opt to treat your body through auricular acupuncture, involving points on the ears only or in combination with points on the rest of your body. This is particularly helpful in reducing stress and addictive behaviors.

We prefer to dim the lights, play light music, and encourage you to relax while you lie there for anywhere from twenty to thirty or so minutes.

Many people assume the needling will hurt, but it is relatively painless. You may feel a pinching sensation for a few seconds in certain points as the needles are inserted, but that feeling diminishes quickly, and if you remain calm and still, you will feel fine.

There are no negative side effects following a treatment, only a sensation of calm. And although an inexperienced or inept acupuncturist can cause infection, bleeding, bruising, or even organ puncture, and if the wrong points are used the effects can be opposite to your treatment goals, these occurrences are fewer than one in ten thousand. But you must check out your acupuncturist's credentials. With an experienced, licensed practitioner, acupuncture is a very safe procedure. Linda, the patient who delivered a healthy baby girl after eleven years of infertility and two unsuccessful IVF cycles, says, "I would recommend acupuncture to anyone with a hormonal or ovulation problem. I feel it not only helped with the FSH, it also helped with all the hormones that are necessary to make my eggs what they should be. It really got my body ready."

"Forbidden Pregnancy Points"

Twenty-four points are called the "Forbidden Pregnancy Points" by acupuncturists because if they are stimulated on a pregnant woman, the pregnancy can be terminated. For this reason, your TCM practitioner must be cautious and not give you treatments if it's possible that you have conceived. If you are also using ART strategies such as IVF treatments, you must make sure your acupuncturist and your fertility doctor communicate with each other.

Acupressure

Acupressure is much less powerful, although the underlying theory of healing is similar to that of acupuncture—locating energy blockages and applying pressure over specific points in order to help free those blockages and promote proper energy, blood, and lymph flow to restore balance, good health, and fertility. Also known by its Japanese term, *shiatsu*, acupressure is accomplished through the fingers. While it is more pleasurable to have someone work on you, you can also perform acupressure on yourself anytime, at your convenience, and it is free. In chapter 10, you will learn easy, step-by-step instructions on how to perform simple acupressure treatments on yourself to boost your reproductive health.

Finding an Acupuncturist and Combining Treatments

In some states, medical doctors can get a license to practice acupuncture after taking a three-hundred-hour-plus course. However, this simply is not enough time to learn everything a practitioner needs to know about this complex healing art—particularly when it comes to treating infertility. Mary F. Bochichio, president of the Florida State Oriental Medicine Association, once likened the limited physician's course to "taking a weekend in surgery."

Non-M.D. acupuncturists must train and practice over several thousand hours at an approved TCM training institution, and then pass rigorous exams to receive state and national board certifications. Many M.D.s who practice acupuncture continue training after receiving certification. Check if your medical doctor/acupuncturist has done this, and particularly if this training is in TCM and fertility. Otherwise, you may be better off seeking out a non-M.D. acupuncturist. In any case, check out any practitioner's qualifications with the American Academy of Medical Acupuncturists and other groups listed in the appendix to this book. Be aware of the following points:

- Your best bet may be an acupuncturist affiliated with a major academic medical center or clinic. Again, at minimum, make sure your acupuncturist is licensed by state and national boards.
- Be sure to tell your conventional fertility doctor that you are interested in trying acupuncture before undergoing treatments. Certain conditions, such as those requiring surgical intervention, may preclude this option for you.
- If you are also undergoing ART, make sure that your reproductive specialist and your acupuncturist have a working relationship and are aware of each other's treatment plans.
- Be sure your reproductive medical specialist knows about any TCM herbs you are taking. Chapter 9 lists and describes herbs a practitioner might recommend as part of your treatment, as well as those you should avoid if there's a possibility that you are pregnant.
- Since some of the acupuncture points that stimulate ovary function are the same ones that can cause miscarriage, you can see that acupuncture, like Western an-

tibiotics or surgery, is strong medicine. We may not know exactly how it works or why, but we do know that this ancient practice is neither hocus-pocus nor primitive. It is a complex and coherent system of thought and practice that has been developed over the course of millennia, and it continues to be subjected to critical thinking and clinical practice. Here in the modern West, traditional Chinese medicine is proving its tremendous powers to protect health, heal an ever-broader spectrum of conditions, and effect lasting change, including helping many people move from conditions of infertility to fertility.

Chapter 3

Getting to Know Your Reproductive Anatomy: The Western and Eastern Perspectives

In our practice, we find that age is a key reason why people are experiencing fertility issues in this modern age. Men and women have spent their twenties developing careers and professions, after which they marry and attempt to reproduce at a later and biologically less optimal age.

This is particularly true for women. Women are born with a finite number of eggs, and as the reproductive years tick away, the number and quality of those eggs decrease. The fertility of women ages thirty to thirty-four is 14 percent less than that of women ages twenty to twenty-four, and for women ages thirty-five to thirty-nine, the fertility rate is 31 percent lower. In women over forty, the percentages drop even more sharply.

As a woman you are biologically programmed to reproduce when you begin menstruating, anywhere from ages twelve to sixteen. When you start menstruating, it means you are ovulating. Biologically, you can begin reproducing—just like our animal cousins that often become pregnant immediately after becoming fertile, that is, when they first ovulate. Of course, few women in our modern society deliberately start reproducing in their early teens, because the optimal sociological time to have a family can be age thirty or later. These days, social and biological reproductive peaks simply do not coincide. Good, solid statistics are telling us that when it comes to reproduction, we are diverging more and more from what we're meant to be doing, at least biologically speaking.

So our culture has gradually deferred the age at which we marry and reproduce over the past fifty years or so, but our biological programming hasn't shifted for millions of years. Women have not started to menstruate at thirty. In fact, women are menstruating at increasingly younger ages than ever before because, among other factors, they are better nourished, so their bodies mature earlier. Hormonal additives in our food and environment may also contribute to earlier onset of menses.

Pregnancy depends not only on sperm managing to fertilize an egg, but also on the fertilized egg successfully implanting in the lining of the uterus, the endometrium. In older women, the hormonal surge that is key to successful conception and implantation of the fertilized egg in the uterus is either no longer present or severely diminished. Age, however, is only one factor that can cause infertility.

Before we discuss how to overcome various fertility obstacles, we want to describe the female and male reproductive systems.

THE FEMALE REPRODUCTIVE SYSTEM: THE WESTERN PERSPECTIVE

In Western medical terms, the hormonal chain of command, the endocrine system, is a complex of glands, organs, hormones, and other chemicals that controls reproduction and virtually every other body function.

Like other alternative and complementary health practitioners, I view the hormonal chain of command as something more. It binds together your psycho-neuro-endocrino-immune systems—in other words, your entire mind-body complex. TCM practitioners, along with all alternative medical doctors, believe that even the slightest imbalance or disruption anywhere in the hormonal chain of command can impair fertility. Of course, your fertility is governed by your menstrual cycle. And that cycle is connected to virtually every aspect of the complicated endocrine system in which a carefully choreographed series of hormonal signals sent out by glands and organs ensures that your body functions smoothly. It takes only a few players involved in the hormonal chain of command to fall out of step for hormonal irregularities to occur in your menstrual cycle and impair your fertility.

Just like ovulation and the fertilization of an egg, implantation of the fertilized egg is a complex and delicate process that involves precisely timed signals from the hormonal chain of command that tell an ovary when to release an egg because the uterine lining is ready to receive it. The window of opportunity is brief and fleeting. The egg must be receptive to the endometrium, and the endometrium must be receptive to the egg. The process of implantation and connecting to the mother's blood supply is so vulnerable that studies estimate from 30 to 90 percent of embryos fail to implant themselves in the uterine lining. In other words, those embryos are lost even before pregnancy is noticed, because they are shed in the next menstrual period.

THE HORMONES AND THEIR GLANDS

- Hypothalamus gland. The hypothalamus gland "sits" in the midbrain, under the limbic area and kicks off the hormonal chain of command after receiving signals from the limbic part of the brain that tell it to release certain hormones. Once the hypothalamus knows what is has to do, it sends its own hormonal instructions down to the pituitary gland, the endocrine system's master gland.
- Pituitary gland. After getting a message from the hypothalamus gland, the pituitary gland sends its own hormonal signals to other organs and glands—the ovaries, the adrenal glands, and the thyroid gland—in the hormone system.
- Neuropeptides. Neuropeptides are chemical messengers created by the nervous system to carry nerve impulses, including the signals set off by the endocrine system, everywhere in the body.
- Ovarian hormones. Ovarian hormones include estrogens, progesterone, testosterone, and DHEA (dehydroepiandrosterone) and they stimulate a response that ensures that the rest of the body—including the lungs, heart and blood vessels, and bones—functions normally.

Within this chain of signals, each gland or organ is stimulated to secrete its own specific hormone, or group of hormones, in order to create changes in particular parts of the body. Each hormone stimulates a specific target area in the brain and the rest of the nervous system.

Hormones affect your entire genital area—the vagina, the bladder, the lower gastrointestinal tract, and especially your ovaries and uterus. Each month, your uterus prepares for the possibility of a fertilized egg by building up the uterine lining. This buildup of the endometrium is caused by surges in certain hormone levels, much in the same way that fertilizer causes grass to grow rapidly and thick. If conception doesn't occur—that is, if sperm does not penetrate an egg—the thick, cushiony uterine lining is shed as a monthly menstruation.

- Hormone-receptor sites. Hormones are able to do essential work because of membranes that line each and every cell of your body. These membranes contain receptor sites for specific and appropriate hormones. The receptor site for each cell is designed to fit only the right hormone, just as a key fits only a specific lock. Once the right hormone has unlocked the receptor site on a cell's membrane, it goes through that membrane to enter the cell's interior, called the cytoplasm, which contains the nucleus or "command center" of the cell.
- Hormone-receptor complex. Another membrane surrounds the cell nucleus that the hormone must pass through via another specific hormone site in order to enter the cell nucleus. Once that happens, a hormone-receptor complex is created. The hormone-receptor complex then creates a protein messenger that sets off certain events in a particular body part.

Of course, one of the hormone chain of command's greatest feats is the menstrual cycle and reproduction. Let's take a look at what happens every month.

THE MENSTRUAL CYCLE

Day One. Day one of a "normal" cycle starts at the end of your menstrual flow. Estrogen and progesterone levels are at their lowest, monitored by a system that continuously checks hormone levels in the bloodstream. The pituitary gland responds to low blood levels of estrogen—as well as to stimulation by GnRH, a gonadotropin-releasing hormone secreted by the hypothalamus gland—by increasing production of FSH. Increased levels of FSH stimulate specialized cells within the ovarian follicle to produce more estrogen. Actually, production is being stimulated for three different human hormones that are grouped together as "estrogens":

- Estradiol. Also known as E2, estradiol is the principal estrogen hormone and the most abundant type during the so-called reproductive years.
- Estrone. Also known as E1, this estrogen is usually interchangeable with estradiol and is equally strong.
- Estriol. The weakest of the estrogens that occur naturally in your body, estriol is most abundant during pregnancy, and it seems to be a biological end product of the two stronger estrogens.

Day Two. FSH sent by the pituitary gland stimulates theca cells in the ovaries to produce more estrogen. As theca cells mature, they produce increasing levels of estrogen. As you approach your time of ovulation—when an ovary releases an egg—blood levels of estrogen keep rising, setting off signs and symptoms of ovulation. One sign is increased mucus secreted by the cervix, the opening to the uterus, at the back of the vagina. That mucus also becomes stickier and "stretchable." If you place a small amount of this cervical mucus between two fingers and then draw them apart, the mucus stretches without breaking. This is called the Spinnbarkeit effect and is used in family planning to detect the approach of ovulation, when a woman is fertile.

Midpoint. As your cycle approaches its midpoint, estrogen levels are still rising. Ovulation usually occurs on day fourteen or so, but it can actually happen anywhere from day three to day twenty-one. Upon ovulation, the pituitary gland releases a pulse of luteinizing hormone, also known as LH. Meanwhile, FSH is still stimulating the ovary, and several ovarian follicles—the egg "sacs" that contain a premature ovum—are developing. Every woman is born with approximately a million immature eggs in her ovaries, and, unlike with men, who continue to produce sperm through their lifetimes, that initial allotment decreases throughout her lifetime.

As the time for the mid-cycle surge of LH approaches, a single follicle releases the mature egg for that month, and the other follicles regress, getting out of the way, as it were, of the victorious follicle, even though they are unlikely to be stimulated ever again.

At this point, "the follicle of the month" is still under the direction of LH, which now stimulates the follicle to release its egg, the ovum, into the abdominal cavity. Though that tiny egg can land anywhere, it can also be detected by the fimbria, the fingerlike projections at the ends of the fallopian tubes that scoop it up and send it down the length of the fallopian tube. No one really knows just how all this is accomplished.

Fertilization normally takes place within the fallopian tube, so whenever transport of the egg is delayed for any reason, the chances greatly increase for an ectopic, or tubal, pregnancy. If the fimbria don't grasp the egg and it drops deep into the abdominal cavity, other problems can result, including a rare but dangerous pregnancy, in which the developing fetus attaches to the intestinal wall and creates an abdominal pregnancy with potentially devastating effects for both mother and fetus.

After the egg has been picked up by the fallopian tube, the empty follicular sac in the ovary converts itself into a progesterone-secreting organ called the corpus luteum. The corpus luteum now produces progesterone to balance the effect of estrogen in the uterus and prepare the uterus to accept and nurture the fertilized egg. It is the body's balancing act between progesterone and estrogen in the uterus that allows a fetus to develop in the uterus and become a child.

The Second Phase. Estrogen signaled your uterus during the first part of the cycle to build up its lining. During the second half of the cycle, the rise in progesterone blood levels signals the uterine lining to stop growing and also stimulates the cells of the lining to differentiate so they can create the right environment to nurture a fertilized egg. This action continues until approximately the twelfth week of pregnancy, when the placenta is developed enough to take over the nurturing job. If there's no pregnancy, the corpus luteum continues producing progesterone for approximately two weeks of the cycle, until it stops functioning and becomes what is called the corpus albicans. This second transformation causes progesterone levels to plummet, which signals the built-up uterine lining to slough off as menstrual flow. Menstrual flow usually occurs on day twenty-eight of the cycle, but many women experience normal cycles that are substantially shorter or longer. Once the flow ends, we are back to day one, and the entire menstrual cycle repeats itself again.

Other major players in the menstrual cycle and pregnancy include the pituitary gland, which also stimulates the adrenal glands, and the thyroid gland, which also produces and secretes ACTH (adrenocorticotropic hormone) and TSH (thyroid-stimulating hormone). All these hormones are important to your menstrual cycle and fertility because they help maintain a healthy balance between estrogen and progesterone secretions.

DISRUPTIONS IN THE HORMONE SYSTEM: THE WESTERN PERSPECTIVE

Most physicians understand that your reproductive system is so complex and sensitive that it can be easily disrupted. Not every doctor is aware, however, that the hormone system can be thrown off even by extremely subtle influences, some of which are still unknown to medical science. For example, a well-known phenomenon confirmed by many studies occurs whenever a group of women live together, such as in a college dormitory. In these instances, a "dominant" female controls the menses of the other women. At first, the "follower" women believe their periods are irregular. Eventually, they realize that all their cycles have come to coincide with the cycle of the "dominant" female. Pheromone production may be the reason for this phenomenon: the "dominant" female produces the most powerful pheromones, chemicals that stimulate the olfactory nerves in the brain and enable you to detect smells. These pheromones also stimulate the brain's limbic system, the hypothalamus, and the pituitary—all of which play important roles in controlling the phases of the menstrual cycle and fertility.

Any number of problems can disrupt your fine-tuned reproductive system. If the nuclear membrane of a cell is healthy, a hormone can enter through its appropriate hormone-receptor site in the lining and reach the cell's command center. But if either the outer membrane or the nuclear membrane is unhealthy, the hormone cannot get inside to do its work. Such poor lifestyle choices as an unhealthy diet, too little rest, inability to cope with stress, or pollutants, can interrupt this process, making you vulnerable to a wide spectrum of disorders associated with hormonal dysfunction, including infertility.

The interplay between several glands is so precise that levels of hormonal secretions are measured in units known as picograms, a trillionth of a gram, and nanograms, a billionth of a gram. Even disturbances at the nanogram or picogram level can create problems. However, despite this extreme sensitivity, our bodies usually do manage to function as they should.

MALE REPRODUCTIVE ANATOMY: THE WESTERN PERSPECTIVE

Among the most breathtaking wonders of the human body is the way the male and female reproductive tracts echo and complement each other in form and function. Like the female reproductive system, the male reproductive system depends on the hormonal web to produce sperm, the man's main contribution to the creation of new life. Even the complex chain of hormonal cues that keeps male reproduction functioning involves hormones almost identical to those involved in the female reproductive cycle. The main difference is that in women the hormonal cycle repeats itself over and over, in an ongoing monthly loop, whereas in males the cycle is continuous, with no beginning, middle, or end. A woman's reproductive cycle changes dramatically over her lifetime and comes to a close during menopause, when she's run out of viable eggs and no longer experiences the hormonal surges that allow a fertilized egg to implant in the uterus. Her partner, on the other hand, has no significant time limit on semen and sperm production. While women are born with their lifetime quota of eggs and begin losing them almost immediately after birth, men's testes churn out millions of sperm on a daily basis for nearly a lifetime. And unlike the female reproductive system, located mostly inside the body, the majority of the male reproductive system is composed of external structures, including the penis, the scrotum, and the testicles.

Let's take a look at the major parts of the male reproductive system:

- Penis. The male organ used during sexual intercourse is made up of the root, which attaches to the abdominal wall, the shaft, and the glans, or head of the penis, which is the cone-shaped part at the end of the shaft. If a man is uncircumcised, he also has a foreskin, a loose layer of skin that covers the penis when it is not erect. The opening of the urethra, which transports both urine and semen, is at the tip of the glans.

The penis consists of three circular chambers composed of spongelike tissue that fills with blood when a man is sexually aroused. This allows the penis to become erect and rigid so it can penetrate the vagina during intercourse. When the penis is erect, the flow of urine is blocked so the man can ejaculate semen during orgasm.

- Scrotum. This loose pouch of skin hangs behind the penis and contains the testicles, or testes, along with nerves and blood vessels. Related muscles contract and relax in order to keep the testes away from the body in order to maintain the slightly cooler temperature that protects normal sperm development.

- Testicles. Oval-shaped organs, the testicles are set in the scrotum and secured at either end by the spermatic cord. Most men have two testes, which are the glands responsible for making testosterone, the primary male hormone (although women have testosterone as well). The testicles also produce sperm in coiled tubes called seminiferous tubules. Sperm cells mature in these tubules until they are capable of fertilizing an egg. It takes about two to three months for sperm to mature, after which mature sperm gather on the outer edges of the tubules, like racehorses champing at the bit at the starting gate, eager to be released into the epididymis.

- Epididymis. This long, coiled tube on the back part of each testicle transports and stores mature sperm cells produced in the testes. During the contractions of orgasm, the mature sperm cells are forced into the vas deferens. If no ejaculation occurs, the waiting sperm die and are absorbed into the body.

- Vas deferens. The first of the male reproductive tract's internal organs, this long, muscular tube connects the epididymis to the pelvic cavity and carries sperm through the ejaculatory ducts and to the urethra, the tube that transports urine and sperm outside the body.

• Ejaculatory ducts. These openings are formed by the meeting of the vas deferens and the seminal vessels, and they empty into the urethra.

• Urethra. Urine and sperm travel through this tube; when the penis is erect, urine flow is blocked so only sperm can be ejaculated.

• Seminal vessels. These pouches attach to the vas deferens near the base of the bladder and provide sperm with a fructose-based fluid that gives sperm energy to move.

• Prostate gland. Located below the bladder and in front of the rectum, the prostrate provides additional fluid to nourish sperm and increase the ejaculate. The urethra runs through this gland, which is why a key warning of an enlarged prostate is decreased urinary flow.

• Cowper's or bulbourethral glands. Located along the sides of the urethra, just below the prostrate, these tiny glands emit a clear fluid that lubricates the urethra and neutralizes trace amounts of acidic urine that may be present.

The male reproductive system is charged with the following jobs:

- To produce and secrete the hormones that maintain male reproductive function
- To produce, maintain, and transport sperm (aka the male zygote or reproductive cell) and protective fluid (semen)
- To discharge sperm within the female's vagina during sexual intercourse

There are two primary glands and hormones involved in controlling the functions of the male reproduction system: the hypothalamus, which releases gonadotropin-releasing hormone (GnRH) into the bloodstream every ninety minutes, and the pituitary gland, which is stimulated by GnRH to release follicle-stimulating hormone (FSH) and luteinizing hormone (LH) into the blood, where they are carried to the testes. LH goes directly to Leydig's cells in the testes, which trigger testosterone production to ensure male characteristics and sperm production. FSH goes to Sertoli cells in the testes, which trigger sperm production.

Just as hormone glands must work smoothly along the entire chain of command for women's bodies to work properly, many of the same hormones are necessary for men in order to manufacture high-quality sperm. For example, problems with either the Sertoli or Leydig's cells can cause overly high levels of either LH or FSH or low testosterone. Any or all of these potential problems can cause a low or nonexistent sperm count.

REPRODUCTIVE ANATOMY AND INFERTILITY: THE EASTERN PERSPECTIVE

When you visit our center or any other TCM practitioner, you won't receive a diagnosis such as "ovarian failure" or "polycystic ovarian syndrome (PCOS). Instead of working from the Western model of the endocrine system—the organs, glands, and hormones involved in controlling reproduction, we refer to an entirely different map of the body—the invisible meridians or energy pathways and functional (not anatomic) organs that tie together your entire mind-body system. While TCM does prescribe standard treatment protocols for a range of conditions, Western anatomy and medical diagnoses usually do not enter into the process of building a TCM diagnostic picture of your specific constitution and overall condition. More and more TCM practitioners, though, are including Western biomedical knowledge in their diagnoses, and we certainly take Western diagnoses into account when we are working in conjunction with a conventional fertility specialist. Otherwise, we spend a good deal of time exploring all possible health and fertility-impairing imbalances through a wide range of possible diagnostic signs and symptoms, according to TCM. Your problem may be infertility, but we and other TCM practitioners will check your pulses, look at your tongue, ask about your diet and lifestyle, and use other diagnostic strategies before developing a treatment plan tailored specifically to your particular condition. As you know, diagnosis and treatment are not separate stages within the Chinese healing system; they are intertwined and continually evolve throughout treatment in order to adapt to your condition.

Some TCM practitioners also base diagnosis and treatment on another key philosophical underpinning of TCM healing: Five Element Theory. Five Element Theory combines the concepts of qi and yin and yang with the five elements (wood, fire, earth, metal, and water), and the following other elements:

- The various organ and glandular systems (heart and pericardium, liver, spleen, lungs, kidneys, gallbladder, small intestine, stomach, large intestine, bladder)
- Tissues (tendons, vessels, muscles, skin, bones)
- The seasons (spring, summer, late summer, autumn, winter)
- The environment (wind, heat, damp, dry, cold)
- Tastes (sour, bitter, sweet, pungent, salty)

- Sense organs (eyes, tongue, mouth, nose, ears)
- Emotions (anger, joy, worry, grief, fear)

Other Five Element Theory correspondences include sounds, odors, developmental stages, body types, and directions (south, center, west, north, east) and colors.

Within Five Element Theory, four main check-and-balance relationships that exist between the major organ and gland systems attempt to maintain harmony between the five elements and the parts of your mind-body complex assigned to each element. This means the organ and gland systems of your body not only perform their own specific roles, they also promote health and fertility by controlling excesses and deficiencies in one another's energy. The various acupuncture points along the meridians are determined by complex interrelationships pictured in the Five Element Chart that illustrates how the elements and their corresponding organ systems, emotions, and so on, affect each other. For example, stimulating a fire point on a spleen meridian will also affect a metal point along that same meridian, and by extension, that point will affect another associated organ system, and so on.

Because it is so complex, most TCM practitioners do not use Five Element Theory in its entirety. Instead, we adapt this viewpoint to a more classical TCM view of how disease and dysfunctions such as infertility develop. In the classic style of TCM, the elements of wind, cold, heat, dry, damp, and combinations of those elements are believed to act in the same ways inside your body as they do outside. Simplistically, if you are exposed to more cold than your body can compensate for by warming itself, your qi slows down and obstructions in energy flow and other substances can form. On the other hand, heat speeds up body functions, causing higher temperatures overall or, in specific locations, inflammation and restlessness. Dampness translates as collection of fluids, such as in cases of diarrhea or discharge. Dryness signifies dry skin and dehydration and can be diagnosed by a cracked tongue. Wind refers to obstructions in qi that cause aching or shooting pain.

So we are not so concerned with a mechanical view of your anatomy and fixing the parts that aren't working; we are focused on promoting flow and balance between organs and glands and all the other elements of your system.

Diagnosing and Treating Infertility

Whether we are treating a man or a woman for infertility, we begin by checking overall health to determine if the general condition is yin or yang, internal or external, caused by cold or heat, excess or deficiency, and other factors we've described. We then look for typical qi imbalances that Chinese medicine links to infertility in men and women. These usually appear in any of three organ systems: the kidney, liver, or spleen. We check for those by noting if you have:

- Healthy menstruation, which involves kidney qi, also regarded as vital energy. Once healthy menstruation is restored, general energy and libido improve, and the kidneys (adrenal glands) perform their hormonal functions at peak.
- Liver weakness, which can manifest as a woman's inability to release an egg, or a man's low sperm count. Stress and depression can weaken the liver system, usually by causing stagnated qi. In this way, overwork, prolonged grief, or chronic stress can be severely damaging

to fertility; yet the effects of these negative emotional states are often overlooked. Unblocking liver qi then allows the practitioner to treat the spleen.

- Deficiencies or blockage in the spleen (usually caused by stagnating liver qi) can result in the fertilized egg not implanting in the uterine lining.

The condition of your kidney qi is particularly important, as TCM believes that reproduction is one of the primary functions of the kidneys (including the adrenal glands). The kidneys store the essential qi of the body and are responsible for the growth, development, reproduction, and normal function of all the other organs. Kidney essential qi is passed along from parents to children and thus is necessary to nurture essential qi during childhood so the kidneys can function properly and produce enough essential qi to ensure menstruation and fertility. For women, blood is also an essential ingredient for fertility. Because the spleen, liver, and heart produce and move blood, proper functioning of these three organs is important as well.

Traditionally, TCM physicians believed that if a woman's menstruation was normal, she was fertile. However, as these practitioners came to know that women can be infertile and still have normal menstrual periods, they incorporated modern biomedical understanding of infertility and female reproduction into their practices when treating women unable to conceive or those with other conditions related to reproduction.

In general, TCM regards female infertility as having several causes: kidney yin and kidney yang deficiency; blood deficiency; and blood stagnation (poor flow).

Each type of condition produces different symptoms, and

treatment involves adjustments of acupuncture patterns and herbal remedies not only during each menstrual cycle but sometimes within each of the four stages of a cycle as well. So the focus of treatment changes depending on the cause of the infertility and the stage of menstruation.

Here are symptoms linked to each potential cause of infertility:

- Deficient kidney yin. This condition is shown by light menstrual discharge that is red and without clots; emaciation; weak, aching lower back and legs; dizziness; vertigo; blurred vision; palpitations; insomnia; dry mouth; a red tongue with little fur; and thready, rapid pulse.
- Deficient kidney yang. The symptoms of this condition are prolonged menstrual cycles; little or no menstrual discharge; dull complexion; low back pain; poor libido; leg weakness; very clear urine and unformed stools; a pale tongue with white fur; deep and thready or deep and slow pulse.
- Blood deficiency. This type of condition is also associated with the spleen. In Chinese thought, the spleen transforms food and water and distributes the resulting essence throughout the body. This transformation is the basis for the formation of qi and blood. A weak spleen cannot maintain a foundation for blood formation, and the result is an insufficient blood supply that leaves none for menstruation. Symptoms of blood deficiency include sallow yellow complexion, late menstruation that is pale and scanty, vertigo, dizziness, dry skin, constipation, pain in the lower abdomen after menstruation, a pale tongue, fine, weak pulse.

- Blood stagnation. Stagnant blood can occur where there is qi stagnation or qi deficiency. Because the liver is responsible for the smooth flow of qi, blood stagnation can occur as a secondary symptom of a weak liver. Infertility caused by blood stagnation is characterized by pain; scanty and dark menstrual flow often with clotting, masses, or swelling in the lower abdominal area; depression; premenstrual breast distention; menstrual cramps; irritability; abdominal distension; a slightly purple tongue with thin fur; wiry pulse.

In the following chapter, we'll take a closer look at how to anticipate problems in the reproductive process. We'll start with the conventional Western medical fertility workup, and then reconsider fertility problems from the perspective of TCM.

Chapter 4

Navigating a Conventional Fertility Workup

By now, you are aware that much can go wrong within the intricate complex of the mind-body system that controls fertility. This is why both alternative and conventional medical doctors usually agree that the first step you should take to put all elements in place for a successful pregnancy is for both partners to undergo thorough general health exams to evaluate physical health and screen for possible problems. Since modern-day TCM and quality nonconventional practices should incorporate Western biomedical understanding of the body in their approach to fertility treatment, this is a good idea even if you choose the natural, holistic route to boosting your fertility.

If you have tried to become pregnant for a year without success, you might want your family doctor to give you and your partner a general exam. Although, we practice TCM in our clinic, we ask all individuals who come to our clinic to undergo a full basic workup that includes, at the least, a physical and checks blood pressure, iron levels, blood sugar, urine, and thyroid and other hormonal levels. Other possible issues that should be discussed at this time include dietary factors that can either inhibit or increase fertility, and the need to eliminate tobacco and alcohol use.

If you have reason to suspect there is a problem, I advise you and your partner to be screened for the following additional potential obstacles to a successful pregnancy through what is known as a fertility workup:

- Genetic problems. Depending on your race, ethnicity, and family history, you can be the carrier of a genetic disorder without being affected by it yourself. Examples include sickle cell anemia, which appears in people of African and Mediterranean descent, and Tay-Sachs disease, which affects European Jews and French Canadians. Some diseases are linked to the female X chromosome and are therefore passed on to children from the mother. Other genetic disorders require both partners to be carriers. Some genetic problems can be resolved through tests and genetic counseling, which can also pinpoint fertility issues. For example, if you've undergone repeated miscarriages, the usual cause is issues involving the egg rather than the sperm, but both of you should have your blood checked during genetic counseling, including a karyotype analysis that reveals the structure and number of your chromosomes.
- Rh incompatibility. Eighty-five percent of us are Rh positive, meaning that we have an Rh factor in our blood. The remaining 15 percent are Rh negative. Either condition is fine, but if a father is Rh positive and

a mother is Rh negative, the child can inherit the father's Rh positive factor. If the child's Rh factor does not match the mother's, the pregnancy can be ended or problems can arise during delivery.

- HIV infection. If there's any possibility that either you or your partner has been exposed to the virus that causes AIDS, the time to check is *before* trying to get pregnant.
- Chlamydia. This is a fast-spreading infection in the United States, in large part because it is usually asymptomatic in both men and, often, in women. Unchecked, chlamydia can lead to pelvic inflammatory disease, a primary cause of infertility in women because of the inflammation and scarring it causes. Although this venereal disease can be treated easily with a course of antibiotics (doxycycline, aka Vibramycin, is the drug of choice), experts estimate that chlamydia causes 50 percent of all pelvic infections and 25 percent of all tubal, or ectopic, pregnancies. A test for chlamydia should be part of your annual gynecological exam, and both partners should be tested before trying to get pregnant.
- Gonorrhea. This sexually transmitted disease also does more fertility damage to women than it does to men, but men who are untreated can become sterile. Together with chlamydia, gonorrhea accounts for 80 percent of all pelvic inflammatory disease, and it's possible to be infected with both STDs at the same time. You should know that hormonal contraception increases your susceptibility to gonorrhea.
- Mycoplasma. This asymptomatic bacteria infection can be at the root of unexplained cases of infertility as well

as recurrent spontaneous miscarriages, so it's important to check for it before planning a pregnancy. If untreated, the bacteria can travel to the uterine lining, where they cause a chronic inflammatory condition known as endometritis, which is different from endometriosis, overgrowth of the endometrial lining.

- Genital herpes. Caused by the herpes simplex virus, genital herpes is not curable but is controllable, and many women infected with the virus deliver healthy babies. It is particularly important, however, to rule out a cervical herpes infection before getting pregnant because it can cause miscarriage, stillbirth, and prematurity, as well as brain injury and blindness in an infant.
- Syphilis. Although syphilis is on the decline, it is at epidemic proportions in certain parts of this country. If undiagnosed in a pregnant woman, syphilis can cause stillbirth or a life-threatening infection in her infant.
- Hepatitis B. A viral disease that inflames the liver, hepatitis B is contracted through exchange of blood and sexual activities. There is no cure, but most people who contract the disease recover spontaneously, and a vaccine provides even more protection than barrier contraceptive methods.
- Hepatitis C. Another viral form of hepatitis, this disease is spread mainly through blood exchange, and less so through sexual activities. Hepatitis C can remain asymptomatic for decades before it causes fatal damage to the liver.
- Group B streptococcal disease. Many women have this form of strep and it causes no problems. But during pregnancy or after childbirth, strep B can cause problems, especially if you have a history of STDs, have

given birth previously to children infected with group B, or have a history of premature labor.

- Rubella. You should also be screened for rubella, also known as German measles. If you contract this disease early in a pregnancy, the fetus can be damaged. The doctor needs to check if you were vaccinated for the disease or if you've developed antibodies to rubella through an earlier infection. In either case, your blood can be tested before conception to see if you are immune.
- Autoimmune disorders. A family medical history and blood work can help spot possible autoimmune disorders that lower fertility. Autoimmune disorders occur when your own immune system turns against parts of your body. While most cases are spontaneous, such conditions are often hereditary and include diabetes, thyroid disease, lupus, and rheumatoid arthritis. Thyroid disease, for example, interferes with the hormonal chain of command that is necessary for ovulation and implantation of the fertilized egg in the uterine wall. Even if your thyroid levels test normal, antithyroid antibodies can still be present that may be an issue for your fertility. The presence of specific antibodies that affect coagulation and anti-sperm antibodies are often overlooked as a cause of infertility in couples.
- Acute or chronic diseases. Anything from asthma to cancer means you need to plan carefully before you get pregnant. Some medical conditions that may not affect you now can cause problems if and when you do undergo the dramatic changes of a pregnancy. Of course, the older you are, the more likely you are to develop a chronic health problem.

There are other common conditions you need to consider if you are planning a pregnancy:

- hypertension (high blood pressure)
- epilepsy
- diabetes
- heart disease
- asthma
- kidney disease
- thyroid or other endocrine conditions
- cancer

For example, diabetes and epilepsy can increase risk of miscarriage or birth defects. Heart disease and urinary tract infections may cause premature labor or poor growth of the fetus. Hypertension can cause fetal distress or *abruptio placentae*, in which the placenta separates from the uterus and threatens the fetus's oxygen supply.

You should also be aware that certain medications must not be used during pregnancy because they can harm the fetus. You might need to switch the drugs you are using to treat certain conditions, such as arthritis or ulcers, or alter dose levels. For example, insulin requirements can change dramatically during pregnancy. If you suffer from a chronic or acute medical condition, your medical team should include a doctor who is familiar with how various illnesses can complicate pregnancy.

If you and your partner have been cleared for general and genetic health problems, and you have been unable to have a successful pregnancy after a year of trying, your next step should probably be a focused fertility workup, if only to clear you both for structural problems that must be addressed before either conventional or TCM infertility treatment can be effective.

THE FERTILITY WORKUP

A fertility workup addresses five basic questions:

Are you ovulating regularly?
What is the quality of your ovulation? (This is determined by your menses.)
Is your partner producing enough viable sperm?
Are egg and sperm able to unite and develop into a fetus?
Is anything preventing the fertilized egg from implanting in your uterine wall and developing normally?

Your Medical History Can Be Key

Always bring a record of your medical history to a fertility workup. This should include your family's medical history so the specialist can screen for possible fertility-related health issues. Your doctor will want to know the following:

- Any previous pregnancies, miscarriages, abortions, or ectopic pregnancies
- Any pelvic surgeries, therapies, or chronic pain
- Any history of cancer therapy that can affect ovarian and testicular function
- Contraceptive history, particularly if it includes hormonal therapy
- If either you or your partner has ever had an STD, suffered from chronic urinary tract infections, unex-

plained bladder pain, or other chronic diseases or conditions

- If either of you is taking medications
- If either of your mothers ever took the miscarriage drug DES (diethylstilbestrol), which can cause reproductive organ abnormalities in offspring
- Lifestyle factors, including nutritional habits and possible exposure to toxins from the outside environment and your home (such as from secondhand cigarette smoke)

In fact, when we are performing a TCM diagnosis, many of these same points are among the questions we ask. The most likely starting place of a conventional fertility workup could be a semen analysis for your partner. It makes more sense to begin by checking if he is sterile or "sub-fertile" (has a low sperm count, for example) than by launching a series of invasive, painful, and expensive investigations on you.

At minimum, a fertility workup should include a semen analysis (sperm test), documentation of ovulation (to prove it's happening), the measuring of blood hormonal levels (levels on day two or three of your cycle of follicle-stimulating hormone and estradiol) to confirm ovarian reserve, an ultrasound of the uterus and ovaries (to rule out endometriosis and other problems), and a hysterosalpingogram (HSG), a test that also evaluates the fallopian tubes and the uterine cavity.

YOUR PARTNER'S (THE MAN'S) FERTILITY WORKUP

Most experts estimate that males contribute equally to any couple's fertility challenges, and if a practitioner suspects that your partner has a reproductive problem, particularly if it's structural, he should be referred to a urologist. The urologist should have an interest or specialization in male infertility and be fully informed on the possible ways of boosting sperm production and quality.

There are many different possibilities to be explored when a man sees a doctor for possible fertility issues.

Medical History

Your partner's present medical history is most important, including exposure to toxic substances that can impair sperm production and quality. Probably the most toxic threat to sperm quality and production is cigarette smoke, whether it's first- or secondhand. Smoking not only causes cancer and vascular disease, it is also the number one risk factor for erectile dysfunction, which is common in the thirty-to-fifty age group. Studies also show that smoking lowers sperm count and motility. Smoking even lowers chances of success for in vitro fertilization when either the man or woman smokes, even more so if both smoke. There's also evidence that if your partner is smoking at the time of conception, the child has an increased risk of developing the cancer known as lymphoma.

Other possible toxins include medications, drug use, and toxic chemical or metal occupational exposure. Though few medications are known to impair sperm production or quality, any medication can have that effect on a particularly sensitive individual, so your partner's doctor will want him to cut down on meds, if possible. For example, an overweight man who does not exercise and is on an antihypertensive medication may be able to go off that drug if he loses weight and follows a regular exercise program. On the other hand, an insulin-dependent diabetic cannot get off his insulin without jeopardizing his health. If your partner is about to be treated for cancer with chemotherapy, it is best to bank his sperm before he begins treatment and not try conceiving through natural means during the treatment. A class of compounds known as calcium channel blockers (used to treat angina pectoris or chest pain, high blood pressure, migraines, brain aneurysms, and other complaints) can impair sperm's ability to fertilize an egg, even though it doesn't seem to affect sperm count or motility. Antidepressants do not affect sperm count or quality, but they can adversely affect ejaculation. Even some lubricants can interfere with sperm. Olive oil is actually the best—and cheapest—lubricant, but there are also commercial lubricants on the market designed not to interfere with sperm.

I and other fertility doctors want to know these things about your partner's sexual and development history as well:

- Whether or not both testicles descended into the scrotum when he was born
- The age at which he went through puberty
- How many sexual partners he's had
- If he's experienced problems with ejaculation or impotence
- If he's fathered a child with another woman
- If he's been treated for a sexually transmitted disease

Plus, we want to know about other lifestyle factors:

- If he takes frequent saunas or hot tub baths
- If he smokes cigarettes or marijuana
- If he's taking any medications
- If he's had a fever in the past three months, ever had mumps (which can inflame the testes), or ever had surgery to the pelvic area

After taking your partner's medical history, the next step is a medical exam that checks for the following:

- General appearance, including such secondary sex characteristics as facial and body hair distribution, physical build, deepness of voice
- Height and weight
- Fat deposits around the breasts (gynecomastia)
- Blood pressure, urine, and reflexes
- Thyroid enlargement
- Irregularities in the penis
- Irregularities in the testes
- Tenderness or swelling in the epididymis that could indicate infection
- Varicoceles around the testes (similar to varicose veins) that reduce sperm count and motility
- Swelling or inflammation in the prostate gland and seminal vessels
- Normal sensation throughout the external genitalia

The Semen Analysis

A man's sperm production declines very slowly over the years, unlike the sharp decline of egg number and viability that occurs in women. In other words, men don't have to watch a biological clock—they don't have to rush to conceive before a certain age—because even very elderly men can become fathers.

Like many people, you may believe that low testosterone is a cause of male infertility, but it's rarely a factor. However, testosterone therapy may impact negatively on sperm production and is therefore not a fertility treatment for men.

A home semen test called FertilitySCORE offers two kits to check sperm quantity in a general way. But this test doesn't reveal anything about motility, quality, or shape—and it's far less accurate than a laboratory test.

In a laboratory sperm test, the doctor asks your partner to provide a semen sample, which can be collected in the laboratory or at home, to analyze for sperm levels and quality. In order to ensure that the sample provides accurate information, your partner has to avoid ejaculating for two to three days before giving the sample. If he does it at home, he should collect the sample in a clean container, keep it at body temperature by tucking the container into the waistband of his pants or under his arm, and make sure the sample arrives at the lab within one hour—half an hour is even better!—before the sperm begins to deteriorate.

Wait to test your sperm for at least four months after a course of medication, such as antibiotics, because it can take that long to recover your normal sperm count. You can help your partner reach orgasm, but oral sex is okay only if you use a non-lubricated condom, because your saliva and vaginal mucus can interfere with test results. Do not collect semen in a regular condom; use a special condom called a semen collection device (SCD). Avoid using lubricants because they may poison the sperm.

The lab will check the sperm sample for the following:

- Color, appearance, and odor to rule out infections
- Coagulation and liquefaction to rule out problems with the seminal vesicles and prostate
- Volume, to rule out such problems as duct obstructions, semen production, overactivity of seminal or prostate glands, or overly frequent ejaculation. However, low volume can be caused by various other factors, including your partner's discomfort with collecting sperm in a laboratory setting. Low volume by itself will not prevent conception unless it is accompanied by other male infertility factors.
- Ph, to ensure semen is slightly alkaline, not overly acidic or alkaline, which indicates infection or inflammation in the prostate or seminal vesicles
- Viscosity, because overly thick or sticky fluid also indicates possible infection
- Concentration of sperm, normally between 20 and 120 million per milliliter of semen
- Motility, to check the sperm's ability to swim. Low motility can be caused by a number of factors. Normal means that at least 50 percent of the sperm move.
- Morphology, to check for the oval head, cylindrical middle, and long, tapering tail that characterizes healthy, mature sperm. The shape of the sperm can be measured a number of different ways, but most studies

find that the shape of sperm has little to do with its genetics or the outcome of a pregnancy. Some people believe the reason sperm is "washed" during intrauterine insemination (IUI, in which your egg is fertilized, then placed in your uterus) is to select genetically superior sperm, but this is not true. Sperm is "washed" to remove the protective membrane coating the head and allow it to penetrate an egg and to reduce the amount of seminal fluid so sperm is concentrated in a small enough volume of fluid to place inside the uterus. The uterus may expand to hold a baby, but during insemination it can hold only a tiny volume of fluid. Some sperm-processing procedures select only motile sperm, but no sperm-washing procedure can select "superior"-quality sperm. There are two standards for what is considered normal morphology of sperm (that is, normal form: not missing a tail, or having two heads). The World Health Organization standard is at least 50 percent normal morphology.

- Clumps of sperm, indicating either sperm antibodies that form as a result of infection or the sperm antibodies that hinder motility
- Infections, detected through culturing seminal fluid
- White blood cells, indicating infection
- Ability of sperm to penetrate cervical mucus, checked through the mucus invasion test
- Crossover sperm invasion test on another female's egg as another way to determine if the problem is with you or your partner

Sperm changes so dramatically from day to day that at least three sperm tests should be performed. In addition, the spectrum of what is normal for sperm is so wide that the parameters for "normal" are minimal. Sperm has to satisfy all three criteria for two out of three tests in order to receive an overall "normal" rating. But please realize that these are minimal conditions that are considered necessary, and they are not always enough to guarantee your partner's sperm isn't contributing to the infertility problem. A man's sperm can be ranked as "normal," but semen analysis is a very rough test. It's like the college applicant we discussed in chapter 1. Just because his grades, scores, and interview are outstanding, there's no guarantee he will be admitted or a good student. Do not be discouraged, though, because there are many ways to enhance sperm quality that we will discuss in later chapters.

If any sperm test results are abnormal, the test should be repeated at least twice to rule out the impact of such factors as fevers and infections that can alter a man's sperm for months. Tests also need to be repeated because every man's sperm count fluctuates up and down on a day-to-day, week-to-week, and month-to-month basis.

Quick Fertility Fixes for Your Partner

Although sperm tests are given multiple times in order to account for temporary changes in sperm quality and production, some very simple adjustments can correct this temporary problem:

- Avoid lengthy soaks in a hot tub.
- Avoid tight underwear that holds the testicles too close to the body; switch to loose boxer shorts.
- Get that computer off your lap. A study in human reproduction found that men who use a laptop computer on their laps raise the temperature of their testes by almost six degrees, which may lower sperm count. Earlier research has determined that a boost in only two degrees reduces sperm concentration as much as 40 percent.

If quick fixes such as switching to showers and roomy boxers don't improve sperm count, consider the relatively common condition of varicocele, in which veins around the vas deferens become dilated, much like varicose veins in the leg, causing a pooling of blood in the veins that raises the temperature of the scrotum.

Sperm analyses can pinpoint any problems with your partner that may be acting as barriers to a successful pregnancy. Unfortunately, growing scientific evidence compiled worldwide shows decreased sperm counts in men all over the world, as well as a rise in male reproductive cancers, such as testicular and prostate cancers. We'll explore possible reasons for these phenomena a little later on.

If your partner has diabetes or has had testicular cancer, the doctor also should perform a urine test to check for the presence of semen immediately after he's produced the semen sample. Diabetes or a bout with testicular cancer can cause retrograde ejaculation, when the ejaculate is propelled backward into the bladder, instead of forward into the vagina. This is because diabetes can cause nerve deterioration at the bladder opening, and if a man's testicular lymph nodes have been removed, accompanying nerve damage can prevent the bladder neck from closing properly. There is no conventional treatment for retrograde ejaculation, but TCM can improve the condition in some cases, and a highly successful ART procedure is able to extract live sperm from urine for use in assisted reproduction.

YOUR (THE FEMALE'S) FERTILITY WORKUP

From your first menstruation, you should have been having annual pelvic exams, or more frequently if you're at risk for sexually transmitted diseases and other problems. In any case, I tell all my patients to have a pelvic exam before trying to get pregnant as an important first step to rule out possible fertility obstacles. Your gynecologist will check for signs of illness or dysfunction in the following organs:

- Vagina and its external parts
- Uterus (or womb) and cervix (the opening from the vagina to the uterus)
- Fallopian tubes (which carry the egg to the uterus)
- Ovaries (the glands that produce eggs)
- Bladder (the sac that holds urine)
- Rectum (the chamber that connects the colon to the anus)

Your doctor will also conduct a detailed physical examination, in order to:

- Note your general health and physical appearance
- Record your weight, height, and blood pressure
- Perform a urinalysis test
- Check your heart and lungs
- Note your secondary sex characteristics, including breast development, hair growth patterns, and fat distribution
- Examine your breasts for lumps and check for discharge from your nipples
- Check for lumps and painful areas by applying pressure to certain points on your abdomen
- Examine your vagina and external vaginal organs for structural problems and painful areas
- Examine your cervix and vaginal walls for signs of infection, sores, growths, or abnormal narrowing or erosion of the cervix
- Check for the size, shape, and texture of your uterus, uterine ligaments, and ovaries and to rule out lumps, bumps, or enlargements that don't belong there
- Examine your rectum for unusual growths, bulging, or pocketing
- Take a Pap smear to screen for possible cancer, other cellular abnormalities, and sexually transmitted diseases

Your Reproductive History

An infertility workup should include a detailed medical history that covers some of the points listed earlier for you and your partner, plus points that are particular to you.

Your doctor will ask about your menstrual history because cycle regularity correlates with regular ovulation. He or she will also ask if you've experienced endometriosis and/or pelvic inflammatory disease, and if you've undergone miscarriages and/or abortions.

Contrary to popular belief, your period isn't supposed to come with the same regularity as the telephone bill. Most healthy women find their cycles last anywhere from twenty-one to thirty-five days. It's a rare woman who gets her period every twenty-eight days. Weight loss, stress overload, excessive exercise, and a host of other factors can throw you off schedule or even cause you to skip a period or menstruate twice in one month. Ordinarily, this wouldn't be a problem, but if this pattern persists, it can be a warning sign that ovulation is diminished.

Your doctor will want to know about your sexual history, including contraceptive use, any attempts to time intercourse to your ovulation, use of lubricants or douches, and possible sexual problems with your partner, such as premature ejaculation or inadequate penetration.

Your doctor will gather information about your lifestyle, such as whether or not you smoke, drink, take prescription or recreational drugs, and if you suffer from any eating disorders. He or she will evaluate your general state of health and take a history of any past illnesses and/or surgeries.

Your doctor is also likely to ask about your mother's reproductive history, including how long it took her to conceive and if she had any miscarriages, ectopic pregnancies, or menstrual irregularities. Your doctor may also ask when your mother began to menstruate, and at what age she began menopause.

At this point, if your partner's semen analysis comes back normal, I advise some infertile people—especially those who do not conceive after several months of TCM treatments—that additional tests are needed to check further for possible issues. Female fertility problems usually fall into two broad conventional medical categories: ovulation issues and hormonal issues.

Ovulation dysfunction accounts for approximately 15 percent of infertility cases. Ovulation dysfunction tied to problems with the endocrine system can be tested through measuring blood levels of various hormones. Postcoital tests evaluate sperm-cervical mucus interaction by testing for what happens to your partner's sperm once they're released into your vagina. You can document whether or not you are ovulating through an ovulation prediction kit, through an ultrasound, or by blood tests that measure your mid-luteal progesterone levels. Basal body temperature monitoring that you do yourself by taking your temperature every morning, before getting out of bed, as well as testing your cervical mucus yourself are still effective ways to monitor your menstrual cycle and know when you are ovulating. We'll tell you how to perform these tests a bit further on.

Some ovulation and hormonal infertility conditions:

- Premature ovarian failure (POF). If you haven't had your period for several months, the problem could be excessive dieting or exercising. If you stop those activities for several months and still do not become pregnant, you should be ruled out for premature ovarian failure (POF), also known as premature menopause, a condition that is often misdiagnosed, in part because oral contraceptives can mask the symptoms. Over half the women who develop POF have to see three different clinicians before they are diagnosed, which is accomplished by a combination of your clinical history and two blood tests done at least one month apart to measure FSH levels (since the levels tend to fluctuate naturally). Some women with POF may have menopausal symptoms such as hot flashes and night sweats. Some may not feel anything. The condition is diagnosed by a blood FSH result measuring over 40 mIU/ml in combination with absence of menstruation for one year or more. Many women are in the gray zone where FSH levels are greater than 10 but less than 40 mIU/ml, but they are considered to have diminished ovarian reserves even though they may not yet be in menopause. If you fall into this category, you may experience tremendous difficulty becoming pregnant. Very occasionally, the cause of POF is genetic or a woman has undergone chemotherapy for cancer or an autoimmune condition and the drug therapy damaged the ovarian reserve. Yet for many other women, the reasons for POF are unknown. In many cases, women with diminished ovarian reserve do have egg-producing follicles (menopausal women do not), but the follicles do not respond to the follicle-stimulating hormone. As a result, estrogen production slows. It is important to know that POF is associated with symptoms of menopause and endocrine disorders, including thyroid disease, lupus, diabetes, and rheumatoid arthritis.

- Polycystic ovary syndrome (PCOS). This is a complex endocrine syndrome that involves infrequent menstruation, a tendency toward overweight, high blood sugar levels (tendency toward diabetes), and the abnormal production of the male hormone testosterone, which leads to excess body hair, and infertility. Women with PCOS have various of these symptoms and certainly do not need to have all of them. The hallmark of the condition, which appears on an ultrasound, is multiple small cysts on the ovaries that interfere with ovulation and hormone production. PCOS is also diagnosed by overly high levels of such androgen hormones as testosterone, and high insulin or pre-insulin (IGF-1) levels. Most experts agree that there is a link between PCOS and infertility. The drug metformin, which is used to treat diabetes by increasing the sensitivity of cells to insulin, can be used to restore normal ovulation and fertility to women with PCOS. Acupuncture and TCM-based herbs are also quite useful, resolving a high percentage of such cases within a few months of treatment, and bringing about successful fertility to almost 50 percent of those who are treated.

- Luteal phase defects. In this condition, insufficient blood levels of progesterone prevent a fertilized egg from implanting properly. This can sometimes be addressed by Western medicine as well as with TCM herbs and acupuncture.

- Hyperprolactinemia. This condition is caused by elevated levels of prolactin secreted in the brain; prolactin normally inhibits ovulation only in breast-feeding women. This condition usually needs to be treated conventionally.

There are structural fertility problems as well. Damage to the fallopian tubes, frequently as a result of unrecognized sexually transmitted diseases, is a common structural problem that can prevent sperm from reaching the egg in order to fertilize it. Other structural problems affect the ability of the uterus to nurture a fertilized egg and allow it to develop into a fetus. This damage can be caused by infections, fibroid tumors, endometriosis, or multiple pelvis surgeries. There can also be congenital defects. Some structural problems are treatable through surgery.

The following are less common causes of female infertility:

- Cervical causes. In a small number of cases, sperm cannot pass through the cervical canal either because of abnormal mucus production or previous surgery to the cervix. While intrauterine insemination may be the answer, alternative approaches—including TCM treatments such as acupuncture, nutrition, and herbs—can remedy cases of infertility that are rooted in abnormal cervical mucus production.

• Autoimmune disorders. Autoimmune disorders can also impair fertility. Autoimmune disorders that adversely affect fertility include any condition that involves production of autoantibodies that cause the body's immune system to attack its own tissues. The most common autoimmune condition is Graves' disease, which is usually associated with hypothyroidism (low thyroid function) and production of autoantibodies against the thyroid. Sometimes the blood test for thyroid hormones may be normal and yet the patient is clinically hypothyroid anyway. If you consistently run low body temperatures and generally always feel cold even in warm weather or environments, you should consider whether or not you are hypothyroid even if the blood test thyroid readings are normal. A trial of thyroid medication may be in order.

Other antibodies that cause the immune system to attack sperm as if it were a dangerous foreign body can obviously present problems. Yet other autoimmune reactions can lead to a thickening of the blood, thus reducing blood flow. Lower blood flow can diminish the quality of the uterine lining, as well as reduce flow of nutrients to the ovaries. These conditions either prevent a fertilized egg from implanting or cause repeated miscarriages. The conventional Western medical approach to autoimmune issues is to repress symptoms in the organs and other body parts affected by the disease, often through anti-inflammatory and immune-suppressing medications. On the other hand, TCM and other alternative health practitioners work whenever possible to stimulate and restore the body's own self-healing mechanisms.

- Unexplained infertility. Anywhere from 10 to 15 percent of couples challenged by infertility fall into this grab bag category. Unexplained infertility is defined as the inability to conceive or carry a pregnancy following one year of unprotected sex when medical fertility evaluations have been unable to find anything wrong. Age does not fall into this category, as age itself can be an explanation for infertility.

Recurrent Miscarriages

For thousands of American women, the agony of infertility is not the inability to conceive but failure to carry a fetus to full term. As many as 2 to 3 percent of couples trying to have a baby suffer recurrent pregnancy loss, which is defined in women under age forty as three or more consecutive miscarriages with the same partner. The reality is that 15 to 20 percent of all conceptions end in miscarriage, but no one knows because they occur so early in the pregnancy. And you can take comfort in the fact that even after three lost pregnancies in a row, your chances of a successful pregnancy are still excellent—around 60 percent.

Most miscarriages occur because an embryo has genetic abnormalities that make it unviable, and this can even be true in women who miscarry often. IVF and preimplantation genetic diagnosis help by ensuring only genetically normal embryos are implanted. Other causes of recurrent miscarriages include:

- anatomic abnormalities in the uterus
- immune system diseases

- hormonal imbalances
- blood-clotting problems
- infections
- chromosomal abnormalities in either parent

If your problem is not conceiving, but carrying a baby to full term, it's a good idea to be screened for the following:

- Hormonal factors. You should be tested for your levels of prolactin, thyroid hormones, and progesterone. After treatment, make sure you are retested to ensure that hormonal balance is restored.
- Structural factors. Uterine anomalies and intrauterine defects are often associated with recurrent pregnancy loss. Various visualizing techniques are used to detect these problems. A hysterosalpingogram (HSG, an X-ray that checks the inside of the uterus, fallopian tubes, and surrounding area using a contrast dye injected through a thin tube inserted from the vagina into the uterus) has been the traditional method of evaluating the uterine cavity. Studies show, however, that a sonohistogram (in which saline is injected into your reproductive tract and imaged with ultrasound) provides a lower rate of false-positive findings, avoids exposure to radiation, uses a less allergenic dye than hysterosalpingograms, and can be performed in an office setting to check the shape and size of your uterus and screen for scars and adhesions, polyps, fibroids, or a septal wall (in which part or all of the uterine wall is divided by a membrane or soft tissue). All these possibilities can affect a fertilized egg's ability to implant in the uterine wall and thrive.

- Uterine factor. The lining of your uterus must be thick enough for the fertilized egg to implant. This is done by biopsy of the endometrium on day twenty-one or later of your cycle. If the lining develops slowly or insufficiently, a conventional medical specialist will give you hormonal treatment with clomiphene citrate, HCG, or progesterone for a few cycles, during which time the endometrial biopsy is repeated. An ultrasound can measure if your lining reaches a thickness of ten milliliters or more at mid-cycle, when you ovulate. Some doctors also measure blood flow to the uterus. As you'll discover later, TCM has its own treatments for improving the endometrial lining.
- Chromosomal factors. Tests for chromosal factors can be performed on miscarriage tissue if it can be preserved. In addition, you and your partner may undergo chromosomal testing to screen out translocation of genes, a cause of miscarriage when the normal forty-six genes are present but are joined abnormally.
- Immunologic factors. Abnormal immune response causes your body to generate misguided protective reactions, for example, when antibodies form to attack your thyroid hormones. Other abnormal immune responses cause antibodies to influence blood-clotting mechanisms within the developing placenta, which nourishes the fetus. In some cases, women are "allergic" to their partner's sperm—the immune system blocks the sperm from reaching the egg—because it mistakes that sperm as a dangerous foreign invader and produces antisperm antibodies. If you have the Rh-negative blood type and your partner is Rh positive, you may take a medication called RhoGAM after every miscarriage to

prevent a harmful antibody from threatening your next pregnancy.

Sometimes the problem can be as simple and avoidable as the doctor's failure to perform a thorough pre-pregnancy medical evaluation that includes checking the uterus for structural problems or screening problems with insulin resistance through a simple blood test.

Some medical experts treat women prone to miscarriages with progesterone, a hormone that is necessary for a healthy pregnancy. While others argue that progesterone merely postpones an inevitable loss, new studies suggest that high doses of progesterone can be effective in a small number of patients.

The truth is that many—up to 40 percent—miscarriages are unexplained, and there is no general consensus among the experts on how to handle this challenging fertility problem. One theory proposes that some women miscarry because the immune system fails to recognize and protect a pregnancy. Followers of this theory try two treatments to restore immune function: one, intravenous immunoglobin therapy that uses blood pooled from thousands of donors to regulate immune response, and, two, lymphocyte immune therapy, which uses blood from the woman's partner to prompt her immune system to recognize a pregnancy. However, some fear the lymphocyte treatment causes miscarriage rather than prevents it; studies are ongoing. If you have suffered repeated and unexplained miscarriages and/or have been diagnosed with "unexplained infertility," take heart in knowing that there are many instances in which women rejected as candidates by IVF clinics because of recurrent pregnancy losses eventually experienced a live, healthy birth with TCM or even without any treatment. Many fertility obstacles we've discussed in this chapter can be treated through TCM or even with acupuncture alone. Before we discuss which fertility issues you can treat successfully with TCM, let's take a closer look at possible structural obstacles to fertility that may make surgery your first treatment option.

Chapter 5

When Surgery Is Necessary

If your fertility workups find any structural obstacles to fertility, these should be treated first, usually by surgery. Possible structural problems include correctible anatomical defects and anomalies (which are usually associated with recurrent pregnancy loss), damage to the fallopian tubes, endometriosis, and fibroids. While we as alternative and TCM practitioners are generally not advocates of invasive procedures where they can be avoided, we are not against surgery when surgery needs to be performed.

Surgery may be your only option to address the following structural problems:

- some congenital uterine abnormalities
- tubal damage and adhesions
- Asherman's syndrome

While surgery can be your best option for the conditions below, each of them can also be treated with TCM to enhance or protect your fertility, depending on the severity of your particular case.

- fibroids
- endometriosis
- endometrial polyps

DIAGNOSING AND EVALUATING STRUCTURAL PROBLEMS

If we suspect a patient is suffering from structural problems that may need surgical intervention, we refer the patient to a specialist. If you are referred to a gynecological surgeon, he or she will use any of various following technologies to diagnose and evaluate the above structural problems:

- Hysterosalpingogram fills the reproductive organs with special dye that reveals through an X-ray blockage, scarring, or growths.
- Endometrial biopsy checks the receptiveness of endometrial tissue to a fertilized egg.
- Laparoscopy is performed through a small incision just below the navel, through which a lighted viewing instrument (a tube with a tiny camera) is inserted. Once the abdomen is inflated with gas, the procedure provides detailed information on possible blocks, scarring, or growths. This method, along with cutting devices or lasers, can also be used to remove scar tissue; treat endometriosis and some fibroid conditions; remove ovar-

ian cysts and tubal pregnancies; and open blocked tubes.

- Laparotomy, done through an incision in the lower abdomen in order to inspect the entire abdominal cavity, can also be used to correct some congenital structural problems, remove tumors, sites of endometriosis (implants of uterine lining growing where it shouldn't), or remove scar tissue to free adhesions.
- Hysteroscopy is performed through the cervix to provide the same information as a laparoscopy, as well as detect any anatomical defects. A hysteroscope entering through the cervix also can be used to remove polyps and fibroid tumors, divide scar tissue, and open blocked tubes.
- Sonohysterography screens and evaluates defects in the uterine cavity associated with repeated miscarriages and is particularly sensitive and accurate.

Now, let's take a closer look at the major structural problems that can keep you from becoming pregnant and their possible surgical solutions.

Congenital Uterine Abnormalities

Most congenital uterine abnormalities result from problems in development of the uterus and tubes in the embryo stage. They include a septate uterus (in which the uterine cavity has a wedge-shaped membrane wall dividing the top of the uterus); a unicornuate uterus (basically a half uterus with a connection to only one fallopian tube), a bicornuate uterus (a single cervix with two uterine cavities that may be partially unified), or a didelphic uterus (two cervixes with two smaller-than-usual uteruses and also sometimes two vaginas at the top of the vaginal canal). If you have any of these abnormalities, you may or may not be able to have a successful pregnancy on your own or possibly after surgery (for example, an uni- and bicornuate uterus may not be adequately repaired by surgery to restore fertility). Again, it all depends on the severity of the particular condition.

In addition, there is a host of rare, even unique, possible congenital problems associated with the endometrial lining, cervix, or uterus that can impact negatively on fertility.

Tube Damage and Adhesions

Your fallopian tubes can be blocked so that either an egg can't pass through to meet sperm or a fertilized egg can't travel to the uterus to implant itself. This is a common fertility obstacle, and surgery can remove the blockage. Which type of surgery and how much possibility of success depend on the location and extent of the fallopian tube blockage. Your doctor will suggest any of the procedures described below if you have no other fertility-related problems. A hysterosalpingogram will reveal if either one or both of your fallopian tubes are blocked by scar tissue (adhesions) or if a tube has a buildup of fluid (hydrosalpinx). Surgery also can reverse a tubal ligation that was performed to prevent pregnancy. Also known as having your "tubes tied," a tubal ligation is a sterilization method in which the fallopian tubes are cut and the ends either clamped or tied off so the sperm's path to the egg is blocked. The success of reversing this procedure often depends on your age—the younger you are, the most likely fertility can be restored.

Your surgery will be performed through a small incision in

the navel, a laparoscopy, or through a laparotomy, a small incision made in the lower abdomen. Both procedures allow the surgeon to inspect the entire abdominal cavity for structural problems, endometrial implants, and scar tissue (adhesions) and make appropriate surgical corrections. Many of the procedures that were performed in the past through a laparotomy are now accomplished through a laparoscopy, but your surgeon's decision will depend on what seems appropriate for your condition.

Commonly performed tubal surgeries include the following:

- Tubal reanastomosis. This is typically used to reverse a tubal ligation or to repair part of a tube damaged by scar tissue from infection. In the latter case, the damaged part is removed and the two healthy ends are joined.
- Salpingectomy. This procedure is performed when a tube has developed fluid buildup, hydrosalpinx, that cuts the possible chances for a successful in vitro fertilization (IVF) in half. The part of the tube responsible for generating the fluid is removed and the two healthy ends are joined.
- Salpingostomy. When the end of a fallopian tube is blocked by fluid buildup, this procedure creates a new opening for the part of the tube closest to the ovary that picks up the egg when it's released. Since scar tissue often re-blocks the tube after surgery, salpingectomy is usually the preferred technique before an IVF procedure.
- Fimbrioplasty. This procedure addresses another problem of blockage, when the problem is in the fringed end of a fallopian tube closest to the ovary. It fixes

the blockage there by rebuilding the fringed ends of the tube.

- Selective tubal cannulation. This is actually a nonsurgical procedure, so it's the initial treatment choice for treating tubal blocks that are near the uterus. The doctor uses either a fluoroscope (which uses continuous beams of X-rays to follow movement in the body, including guiding the placement of a surgical tube into the fallopian tube via the uterus) or a hysteroscope (a lighted instrument inserted through the vagina to guide the doctor, along with a cannula that travels through the cervix into the uterus and then into the tube.

The success of any tubal procedure depends on age (especially in the case of reversing a tubal ligation), whether or not there's scar tissue in your pelvis, if diseases are present in the pelvic area, and, of course, your surgeon's skill. Like all surgeries, these procedures carry risks, including: infection; scar tissue, known as adhesions, that bind reproductive organs to each other, to other organs, or to the abdominal wall; and increased risk of ectopic pregnancy.

A hysterosalpingogram may be necessary a few months after a procedure to check if the tube or tubes have remained open and clear. If a year to a year and a half passes without pregnancy, it may be necessary to perform a laparoscopy to take a closer look.

Asherman's Syndrome

In this relatively rare condition, bands of scar tissue join one part of the uterine wall to another, sometimes joining the walls together so completely that the uterine cavity is obliterated. Symptoms include decreased menstrual flow and menstrual and abdominal pain. If this condition goes untreated, menstruation can cease and infertility set in. Causes of Asherman's syndrome include overly aggressive surgical scraping of tissue from the uterine wall (dilation of the cervix and curettage of the uterine lining), intrauterine surgery to remove fibroid tumors or correct anatomical defects, and endometrial infections related to IUD use or an STD. Depending on the severity of the condition, surgery tries to separate the uterine walls and remove the scar tissue. The thicker the adhesions, the more difficult they are to repair because they are more likely to contain blood vessels and some muscle tissue. If there are mild to moderate adhesions, the chance of successful pregnancy after repair is 60 to 80 percent.

All of the above fertility obstacles can be resolved through surgery. While TCM can't correct these conditions, it can be used as a follow-up treatment to correct energy imbalances that caused the problem in the first place so it won't return, as well as to speed recovery and healing.

In some instances, the following structural conditions can be treated through TCM.

Fibroid Tumors

Fibroid conditions are a very common structural obstacle to pregnancy, but only if the tumors are large or numerous enough or positioned in certain ways. Nearly one-third of European American women and half of African American women suffer from fibroid conditions. Although a serious fibroid tumor condition no longer means an automatic hysterectomy, half a million American women have hysterectomies a year, most often because of fibroid tumors. Today, conventional medicine also uses medications and procedures to shrink or remove fibroids while preserving the uterus and ovaries. Many of these medications and procedures, though, can threaten fertility. In many cases, TCM can reduce a fibroid problem to a level where it is controllable and fertility is preserved.

What Are Fibroids? Smooth benign tumors composed of fibrous and muscular tissue—the same tissue as the uterus—that grow in and around that organ, fibroids (also known by the medical term *leiomyomata*) are a mystery. We don't know what causes them; in fact, we don't know what causes any type of tumor. Though their tissue is identical to uterine tissue, fibroids are usually encapsulated by another band of tissue, and grow independently. Their size is usually described in terms of various fruit or the stages of a pregnancy, such as "ten weeks" or "twenty weeks."

Fibroid Symptoms Some women with fibroids have no symptoms, but others suffer from complaints that include lower abdominal pain and pressure, heavy menstrual bleeding, between period bleeding, anemia (and associated weakness and dizziness), indigestion, chronic vaginal discharge, constipation, urinary frequency, bladder irritation and infections, and, of course, infertility and miscarriages.

Types of Fibroids There are four places uterine fibroids grow, thus four types. Each of these four types can create its own problems, and most fibroid conditions include at least two types.

- Subserous fibroids are found on the outer uterine wall and often cause the uterus to grow, usually during menstrual periods, because increased blood flow gives it more nutrients. During menstruation, abdominal bloating and worsening of all other symptoms is typical, as well as pain during intercourse and pain in the back and/or the groin that can shoot down the legs. This type of fibroid can swell a uterus to the size of a watermelon or a "seven months" pregnancy, sometimes putting pressure on adjacent organs.

- Submucosal fibroids grow inside the uterine cavity, where they can cause abdominal cramping severe enough to mimic the pains of childbirth, because the uterus cramps in its attempt to "deliver" the fibroids, as it would a baby. An aborting submucosal myoma (fibroid tumor) means the uterus has actually delivered the fibroid through the cervix and vagina. Not surprisingly, submucosal fibroids typically cause major bleeding problems, with hemorrhaging during heavy, often lengthy periods or upon "delivery." Unfortunately, this type of fibroid condition is the most common reason for complete hysterectomies, and it is the most difficult to heal through TCM or any other alternative healing modality.
- Intramural fibroids develop within the uterine wall—either toward the outside like the subserous type, or toward the inside like the submucosal type. Intramural fibroids therefore can cause the same symptoms as these other types.
- Pedunculated fibroids attach to the uterus by a stalk, and are often mistaken for ovarian tumors because they can look like a large ball on the outside of the uterus when imaged through ultrasound or other visual technologies. When they cannot be clearly visualized, sur-

> gery is usually done to see the problem clearly enough for an accurate diagnosis. As is often the case, location is key in deciding whether or not fertility is affected.

A growing number of physicians, backing away from automatic hysterectomy as the remedy for troublesome fibroid tumors, instead are opting for new, more limited surgical procedures. But these options still yield mixed results, especially when it comes to protecting fertility.

If one of our patients has a fibroid condition, we do not automatically refer her to a surgeon to have them removed. A woman who has a fibroid condition is often able to conceive and bear healthy children if the condition is not severe. This usually means the fibroid tumors are not so large, numerous, or positioned in such a way that they prevent implantation of an embryo and the fetus's full-term development. While conventional physicians tend to view fibroid conditions as the result of genetics and hormonal imbalance, we TCM practitioners conceptualize the problem slightly differently, as rooted in imbalances of fluid and energy anywhere in the mind-body system. In other words, I approach fibroids in the same way that I approach and treat any health problem, by finding and correcting imbalances wherever they are so that the body can self-correct and use its own healing mechanisms to restore health and fertility. While it is extremely difficult to heal fibroids completely, TCM can reduce their size and stop their growth. This means that even if you have a fibroid condition, TCM can reduce its severity to the point where you can conceive and bear a healthy child.

If a patient's fibroid condition resists TCM treatment or is clearly too severe, I will refer that patient to a surgeon who can judge which of the following surgical procedures can be used, always keeping in mind the goal of preserving fertility whenever possible.

- Myomectomy. This procedure involves removing the fibroids only and therefore should not interfere with a woman's ability to have children. It can be done through a "bikini line" incision in the lower abdomen or through laparoscopy (done mostly for subserous fibroids). Yet this surgically conservative operation is more difficult than a hysterectomy, so it must be performed by a highly skilled surgeon who can minimize the threat of negative outcomes, including excessive blood loss, infection, torn uterine lining, perforation of the bowel, or other problems. Once the uterine cavity has been entered, any pregnancy that may follow will require a cesarean delivery because of uterine weakness caused by the surgery. Furthermore, a myomectomy, like any other pelvic surgery, can create or aggravate the hormonal imbalance that may have caused the fibroid condition. Finally, this procedure does not prevent fibroids from growing back.
- Cryomyolysis. This is a procedure, included in newer fibroid destruction techniques, in which the fibroid is destroyed by a probelike instrument that freezes the fibroid's interior.
- Electromyolysis. This procedure also destroys the fibroid's interior via a probe, in this case, by passing an electrical current through it. Again, this is a relatively new and experimental tool that may or may not be successful and only in certain situations at that.
- Laser myolysis. In this procedure laser beams are sent into the core of the fibroid tumor to destroy it.

To sum up, all the above myolysis procedures effectively relieve fibroid growth but often only for the short term. At worst, they can create more problems.

- Uterine artery embolization (UAE). This procedure, used successfully in the past to reduce severe uterine bleeding during an operation, recently was adapted to treat fibroids. It involves passing small particles through blood vessels in the leg that lead into the pelvic area, so that these vessels that are nourishing the fibroids are blocked. Blood flow to the fibroid reduces, causing it to shrink. Embolization techniques don't always work, and because no long-term follow-up is yet available on this relatively new procedure, we don't know how long its effects last or what the negative effects could be.
- Hysteroscopic resection. Some doctors are opting for hysteroscopy to treat submucosal fibroids. A surgeon guides a resectoscope, a wand-like instrument linked to a video monitor and ending in a surgical "loop," through the vagina into the uterus, where the resectoscope "shaves" the fibroid from the uterine wall. Although this option seems less aggressive than a hysterectomy, it is not a benign procedure. Large volumes of fluid need to be instilled into the uterus in order to visualize the fibroid, and problems with fluid absorption are common. Women have actually died from fluid imbalances caused by this procedure.
- Endometrial ablation or resection. This technique destroys the uterine lining, thereby starving the fibroid. And it does not preserve fertility.
- Supra-cervical hysterectomy. A supra-cervical hysterec-

tomy removes only the portion of the uterus containing the fibroids, leaving the rest of the organ intact. This procedure does not preserve fertility, but it does leave most of the pelvic support structure intact, which reduces risk of bladder function impairment and other hysterectomy-linked complications, such as vaginal vault prolapse.

When Does a Fibroid Condition Prevent Pregnancy? With a fibroid that swells the uterus to the size of a "fourteen to twenty-two weeks" pregnancy—a common size—no panel of experts (called in hospitals "the Tissue Committee"), no matter how conservative, would question the decision to opt for hysterectomy. Even if the patient and physician do decide on a hysterectomy, if possible the ovaries or cervix should be preserved, unless there are other mitigating factors.

Unfortunately, no cut-and-dried formula exists for determining that a fibroid is preventing pregnancy or causing miscarriages. There's not even a standard for determining at what size a fibroid or group of fibroids will impede fertility. This is why we will often refer a patient with what seems to be a serious fibroid condition to a conventional medical specialist.

There are two steps you and your medical practitioner need to take to help determine whether or not a fibroid condition is causing your infertility. First, you should rule out other known causes of infertility or miscarriage. And, second, a hysterosalpingogram or the newer and preferred technique of sonohysterography should be performed to detect any congenital uterine defects, as well as provide enough information for your doctor to assess the impact of your fibroid condition on your uterus. If either of those tests or an ultrasound show that your fibroids are not near the uterine cavity, removing them is not likely to affect your fertility.

Again, none of the above surgical procedures ensures that the fibroids will not reappear or regrow, and none is effective for all fibroid conditions.

Other conventional medical methods for shrinking fibroids include GnRH agonists that shrink fibroids by stopping estrogen production and menstruation. These often produce side effects normally associated with menopause, and, of course, they impair fertility. In addition, fibroid growth usually resumes one to three months after the medication is stopped. Other common fibroid medications that also suppress fertility include medroxyprogesterone acetate, a progesteronelike drug, and supplements of male hormones known as androgens that lower estrogen levels and carry possible side effects, including facial hair, voice changes, and acne. Obviously, these are not good options if you are trying to become pregnant.

An Alternative View of Fibroids As alternative and TCM practitioners, we believe that surgery may be necessary to correct fibroids, yet none of the conventional medical options deals with correcting underlying health problems that created the fibroid condition. Many alternative and complementary health practitioners view such rogue tissue growth as fibroids as nature's way of isolating and protecting the body from toxins caused by poor diet, unhealthy lifestyle habits, and environmental poisons that cannot be disposed of through the body's normal elimination processes.

While most medical experts—both conventional and alternative—agree that long-standing disturbances from these factors create the hormonal imbalance that is probably at the root of fibroids and many other infertility-impairing conditions, all we know for sure is that the female hormone estrogen stimulates fibroid growth. Some evidence suggests that progesterone might also stimulate fibroid growth. This theory is supported by the fact that fibroid tissue, just like uterine tissue, contains both estrogen- and progesterone-receptor sites. Medical experts also know that the presence of progesterone-receptor sites in fibroids may actually allow them to shrink.

When used correctly, alternative and holistic healing modalities such as TCM offer practical and effective solutions for addressing the imbalances and dysfunctions that cause fibroids to develop, thereby helping correct the problem for the long term. Increasing numbers of committed health care practitioners and their patients are exploring these options, which include nutritional and other lifestyle changes, herbs, and acupuncture. Later we will describe these alternative fibroid-healing strategies that promote natural hormone balance and increase the chances of a successful pregnancy. It's important to keep in mind that when it comes to fibroids and other hormone imbalance–related conditions, surgery, and fertility, each case has to be decided on its individual factors.

TCM practitioners attribute fibroids and other reproductive issues not just to hormone imbalances but also to the deeper issue of blockages in qi, as well as in fluids. These blockages cause deficiencies and excesses anywhere in the body and are treated with acupuncture, often along with herbs, nutrition, special exercises, and other lifestyle modifications. As you've already learned, the traditional Asian medical view maintains that free flow of qi and fluids through the meridians that tie together the entire mind-body system is essential for optimum health and fertility. So there is no single prescribed TCM treatment that is used for all fibroid conditions. Each patient is viewed as a unique mind-body system in which the causes and locations of imbalances leading to a fibroid condition will vary.

Endometriosis

Until the 1980s, this common cause of chronic pelvic pain was largely unrecognized, and women who complained were generally dismissed as hypochondriacs looking for an excuse from marital duties. Yet approximately 5.5 million women in North America suffer from endometriosis and it's a common affliction for those of reproductive age. Simply put, endometriosis is a condition in which the tissue that lines the uterus, the endometrium, begins to grow in areas outside the uterus. Pieces of uterine lining ranging from small to large can implant themselves anywhere in the pelvic area—on the ovaries, fallopian tubes, intestines, bladder, vagina, cervix, and vulva. Endometrial tissue even has appeared on the lungs, arms, thighs, and elsewhere outside the abdomen. These growths or tumors can cause many problems, including rupturing that causes bleeding, inflammation, scar tissue, and obstructions that impede normal organ function and fertility.

One type of endometriosis affects women who have given birth to a child. In this case, the endometrial tissue breaks through the barrier that protects the muscles in the uterine wall and infiltrates the wall.

Severity of an endometrial condition is measured in stages and by a scoring system.

Stage 1 signifies a minimal problem in which the invading endometrial tissue is thin and fragile.
Stage 2 is still mild but the tissue has infiltrated more deeply.
Stage 3 is classified as moderate.
Stage 4 is the most serious, in which the invading tissue is dense and deeply implanted.

Pain is the number one symptom of endometriosis, although pain is not related to the extent of growth, but to the type of endometrial tumors. Women who have endometriosis usually have regular periods.

What Causes Endometriosis? Possible culprits include "retrograde menstruation," in which some menstrual tissue backs up into the fallopian tubes during menstruation, implants itself in the abdomen, and then grows there because the immune system doesn't take care of the problem. Some researchers theorize that the lymphatic system distributes endometrial tissue from the uterus to other parts of the body, and that this could be a genetic trait. Another possibility is that a woman with endometriosis has retained fragments of her own embryonic tissue that later develop into endometriosis. Other researchers suggest that women with endometriosis may be missing a protein in their uterus, called beta 3 integrin; this can be tested with a timed biopsy of the endometrium. Yet knowing the cause does not affect how endometriosis is treated.

Conventional Diagnosis and Treatment Definitive diagnosis is done through a laparoscopy that determines the presence, location, size, and extent of these growths. Endometriosis, pelvic inflammatory disease, irritable bowel syndrome, and even ovarian problems share similar symptoms, so a laparoscopy is important for an accurate diagnosis.

There is no definitive cure, but conventional medicine treats many women with this condition with oral contraceptives that stop further growth or by inducing a pseudomenopause, which, of course, causes early menopause and impairs fertility. Other therapies include gonadotropin-releasing hormone delivered either through an injection, a nasal spray, a subdermal (just under the skin) implant, or a progestin drug, usually medroxyprogesterone. All these options impair fertility.

Surgery, either through a laparotomy or laparoscopy, removes the growths either through a laser or a cautery that burns them off, or small instruments that cut them off. About 40 percent of the women who undergo surgical removal of endometrial tissue do become pregnant.

Ironically, oral contraceptives are usually the first treatment of choice because they cause the body to enter a false pregnancy. Even more ironic, actual pregnancy can also cure endometriosis; if endometriosis is preventing fertility, however, that is clearly not an option. Women with endometriosis also have a higher risk of tubal pregnancy and miscarriage.

As with other conditions, TCM and other alternative and complementary health practitioners treat this one by taking a deeper look at the patient's overall health and by using strategies designed to promote the body's own self-correcting mechanisms.

As in the case of fibroids, alternative and complementary physicians tend to pin blame on estrogen dominance, an overabundance of estrogen in the body. Some researchers point to environmental toxins, particularly the common chemicals found in our food, water, air, and just about everywhere around us that act as pseudo-estrogens and bind to the estrogen-receptor sites in body cells. When these chemicals acting as false estrogens enter cells instead of the body's natural hormones, they produce new and abnormal hormone-receptor complexes. This information also has been linked to the steadily decreasing rate of animal and human fertility and escalating rates of reproductive cancers.

TCM practitioners build an even more comprehensive diagnostic picture before treatment because, just as they view fibroids, they view endometriosis as rooted in imbalances anywhere in the mind-body system.

Endometrial Polyps A polyp is a small tissue growth that usually has a stem or stalk and can appear on the inner surface of the nose or throat, or in organs such as the large intestine or uterus. Though most polyps are not cancerous, they can become cancerous over time. Again, TCM can correct this condition by rebalancing the mind-body system through acupuncture, possibly in conjunction with herbs, nutrition, and other lifestyle modifications. In contrast, conventional medicine treats uterine polyps that are determined to be a cause of infertility by removing them by a D & C.

YOUR PARTNER'S (THE MAN'S) STRUCTURAL PROBLEMS AND SOLUTIONS

The following equation always holds true: good sperm production plus motility equals better chances of conception. So while most people tend to believe structural fertility obstacles are largely a woman's problem, always make sure all the basic factors necessary for pregnancy are in place, from the standpoint of you *and* your partner.

One common structural problem found in men is a condition known as varicoceles, in which veins around the vas deferens, the duct that carries sperm from the testicles to the urethra, dilate in a way similar to varicose veins. In some men, varicoceles do not impair fertility. In others, these enlarged veins reduce sperm count and motility by causing the temperature in the scrotum to rise, thereby decreasing blood circulation and impairing sperm production. A varicocele is detectable if the doctor feels it; a subclinical varicocele means it can be detected only by ultrasound. Some fertility experts believe that subclinical varicoceles do not affect fertility. If sperm count and motility are impaired and varicoceles are present, I will try TCM to see if the condition corrects on its own, after balance has been restored throughout the mind-body system. Of course, a conventional doctor who diagnoses varicocele as a factor in infertility will likely recommend a surgical procedure called a varicocelectomy, which removes or repairs these enlarged veins.

A varicocelectomy improves reduced sperm levels and motility in about 70 percent of men who have both a detectable varicocele and reduced sperm count and/or motility. Some researchers who've analyzed past studies found little improvement—only 1 percent—in pregnancy rates among partners of infertile men who had surgery to repair varicoceles. Other experts argue that those findings may have been swayed by the poor quality of the studies analyzed. They maintain that corrective surgery to improve blood flow and lower testicular temperature is a good option for men with low sperm counts and motility who also have varicocles.

The following problems can be congenital, which means

your partner was born with them, or they can be caused by disease, injury, or stress. While surgery isn't always the answer, other alternative, fertility-restoring solutions are usually possible.

- Retrograde ejaculation. When the bladder neck doesn't close completely during ejaculation, semen can be forced back into the bladder. This condition is often linked to men who are diabetic or have a history of testicular cancer. In my experience, TCM can work in situations like this, even where conventional medicine has determined the condition can't be cured. If your partner is faced with this situation, and TCM is not able to correct retrograde ejaculation, I'll refer him to a specialist who will retrieve sperm from the urine and use it to inseminate you during your ovulation, a process known as intrauterine insemination. On the day his sperm is retrieved, your partner takes two sodium bicarbonate tablets in order to make his semen more alkaline and protect the sperm.
- Undescended testicles. Babies born with this condition usually self-correct after six or so months, but sometimes the testes have to be descended through surgery. The important point about this condition is that it keeps testicles in the abdomen, where temperatures are too warm for sperm to survive. If untreated, this condition not only causes sterility, it also poses a strong risk for cancer. Even after surgery, your partner may have a low sperm count, so intrauterine insemination may be the solution. My advice is to try TCM first, as it is far less costly and invasive than surgery,

and it always exerts beneficial effects on your overall health.

- Blocked or missing ducts. The sons of women who have taken the anti-miscarriage drug DES are particularly prone to congenital defects that include a missing or malformed vas deferens or missing seminal vesicle that cause low semen volume with low or nonexistent sperm count. The only way around this obstacle is through sperm aspiration, in which immature sperm are surgically removed from the epididymis (where they develop) and cultured in a laboratory until they are mature.
- Hypospadias and epispadias. Both these conditions involve a congenital malformation of the urethral opening, in which the opening appears on the underside of the penis (hypospadias) or on the upper side (epispadias). These conditions don't affect sperm quality, motility, or count, but when sperm is ejaculated, it tends to miss the cervix, through which it can enter the uterus and fallopian tubes. Surgery is an effective option, in which the old opening is closed and a new opening is formed for the urethra.
- Torsion. Injury to a testicle, which can be caused by surgery to repair a hernia or the bladder, can cause it to twist away to protect itself while inside the scrotum. TCM can treat torsion, but it may be necessary to opt for surgery to repair it. The important point to remember is if torsion is left untreated for too long, the testicle or both testes can shrink and atrophy to the size of a pea. In such cases, sterility cannot be reversed.

Now that you are aware of possible structural obstacles to fertility within you or your partner, let's take a closer look in the next chapter at the nonstructural blocks to a successful pregnancy, from both the Western and Eastern points of view.

Chapter 6

Working with Hormone and Immune Issues and Unexplained Infertility: The Western and Eastern Perspectives

In our practice, we try to establish the cause(s) of infertility according to TCM healing principles and then develop a comprehensive therapeutic program that we continually modify to meet the individual's evolving needs. The goal of our TCM-centered therapy is always to treat any fertility problem with healing modalities that stimulate and support the body's self-correcting mechanisms. Through acupuncture, nutrition, herbs, relaxation programs, and other "natural" strategies for strengthening, cleansing, stimulating, and rebalancing, your body can recover optimal function and restore fertility on its own.

In chapters 8 through 11, we'll describe in further detail each of these natural strategies for rebalancing and stimulating your mind-body system's own healing mechanisms. In this chapter, we will focus on major *nonsurgical* fertility issues.

HORMONE IMBALANCE AND FERTILITY

If you and your partner have been cleared for structural fertility impediments, Western medicine, including alternative and complementary physicians, generally looks to hormonal imbalance as a possible cause. As we pointed out in chapter 3's discussion of reproductive anatomy, if any part of the hormonal chain of command (the endocrine system) that controls the ebb and flow of everything from menstruation to sleep doesn't function as it should, your hormones tend to fall out of balance and impair your ability to have a child.

The TCM view also attributes nonsurgical fertility problems to issues of imbalance, although within TCM, the definition of imbalance goes broader and deeper. All disease and dysfunction are rooted in blocks of energy and fluid that can impede free flow anywhere in your complex mind-body system. According to TCM, energetic and fluid imbalances cause areas of stagnation and deficiency that, in turn, keep your organs, glands, hormones, and other parts from functioning as they should.

Imbalances that result in endocrine system problems impede your fertility either of two ways: by interfering with the synchronized hormonal changes that allow the egg to be released from the ovary and signal for the endometrium to thicken in preparation for a fertilized egg, or by interfering with the ability of the fertilized egg to implant itself in the lining of the uterus.

In conventional medical terms, both types of hormonal problems manifest themselves as ovulation or uterine lining issues. Your TCM practitioner will use acupuncture and other strategies in the TCM healing arsenal, while a conventional medical doctor will prescribe drug and/or hormone therapy if you have any of the following issues:

- Elevated levels of prolactin
- Excess of adrenal androgens (male hormones)
- Amenorrhea (lack of menstruation)
- Lack of or infrequent ovulation
- Premature ovarian failure (POF)
- Pituitary failure
- Endometriosis
- Specific glandular disorders
- Premature menopause
- Luteal phase defects
- Polycystic ovary syndrome (PCOS)

FERTILITY AWARENESS (AKA FAMILY PLANNING)

The first step in determining nonstructural causes of infertility is to determine whether or not you are ovulating and, if you are ovulating, at what point in your cycles. As you know, the entire reproductive cycle, including ovulation, conception, and gestation, is controlled by hormones that are released at precisely the right times in precisely the right amounts.

TCM practitioners use the diagnosis techniques described in chapter 2 to determine whether or not you are ovulating, including taking your pulse, looking at your tongue, and questioning you about the quality, frequency, and duration of your menstrual periods. Conventional physicians use medical ovulation-monitoring techniques that evaluate ovulation through detecting the LH (luteinizing hormone) surge in your urine or by vaginal ultrasound. LH is produced by the pituitary gland in both sexes. In men, LH levels remain fairly constant to stimulate the testosterone production necessary to manufacture sperm. In women, however, LH helps regulate your menstrual cycle and egg production, so its levels rise and fall throughout your cycle. A surge in LH indicates ovulation is imminent and you are in your fertile period.

However, even scientific studies show the medical technologies sometimes may not work any better than such "low-tech" methods as basal body temperature (BBT) charts, in which you track ovulation through recording your resting body temperature over a period of time, or the Billings method, in which you determine ovulation periods by noting changes in your cervical mucus. The minor inconveniences of taking and charting your daily basal body temperature and/or monitoring your cervical mucus in order to detect changes that indicate ovulation is taking place, as we tell our patients, are offset by the great advantage of becoming more in touch with your own body, participating in your fertility process, and having almost no cost (just a thermometer).

The point of fertility awareness is to pinpoint the five or so days per month when you are able to become pregnant because you are ovulating. Once you can pinpoint your time of ovulation, you know when you are fertile—for five or so days leading up to ovulation. This gives you the option to time intercourse to this fertile period or, if conventional medical strategies are your choice, to undergo fertility tests and/or fertility procedures that increase your chances of pregnancy.

Timing Intercourse

Sperm has been found in the fallopian tubes as soon as three minutes after ejaculation and is capable of fertilizing an egg for up to three days. Current evidence suggests that the highest probability of conception occurs with intercourse one to two days prior to ovulation, and not the day of ovulation itself. Therefore, once ovulation is detected by any of the methods listed below, it's a good idea to have intercourse that evening and the following morning. In addition, peak sperm concentration occurs after three to five days of abstinence.

Some women are able to figure out that ovulation is about to take place because of monthly bodily changes, including breast swelling and tenderness or pain, increased libido, or a sharp pain on either side of the lower abdomen that signals the egg's release from the ovary. Most women, though, don't experience ovulation symptoms. If you are in that majority, you can increase fertility awareness through the three natural methods for determining when you are fertile:

- Calendar or rhythm method. For centuries, women kept track of their menstrual cycles in order to predict fertility based on this personal history. The rhythm method tracks menstrual period frequency and length over several months at the least, and then estimates fertility based on the fact that ovulation occurs between nine and seventeen days after your period. If you consider the first day of menstrual flow as day one, you can predict your probable ovulation time by subtracting fourteen days from your typical menstrual cycle length. For example, if your menstruation cycles are typically thirty-three days apart, subtract fourteen from thirty-three for an anticipated ovulation on day nineteen. However, this method clearly depends on regular cycles. If yours are irregular, the rhythm method is probably not for you. Better choices for predicting your ovulation are tracking your basal body temperature and cervical mucus throughout your cycles.

- Basal body temperature (BBT). Your basal body temperature is the lowest body temperature you experience during a day. Usually this occurs in the morning, just after waking up and before getting out of bed. The hormones that control your menstrual cycle also cause bodily changes; changes in your basal (resting) body temperature counts among those changes. Science has discovered that your lowest basal body temperature occurs a day or two before ovulation. Your highest temperature is one to two days after ovulation. If you measure and chart your basal body temperature every morning before rising, after a few cycles, you will be able to estimate your time of ovulation.

How to Take Your Basal Body Temperature

For several months, just before you get out of bed to eat, drink, urinate, or bathe, take your temperature orally or rectally with a thermometer that has markings in tenths of degrees (0.1). Keep the thermometer in a convenient place, just by your bedside, and shake it down to 95°F each night or just after using it in the morning. Do not shake it down in the morning before taking your temperature, as it's important to avoid any activity to get an accurate reading. Use the same location for insertion (mouth, anus, or armpit) and use the same thermometer each time.

Leave the thermometer in place for a full five minutes. Record your basal body temperatures over time on a chart. After a few months, you will know when you're ovulating because your basal body temperature increases by 0.4°F and stays high for about a week. To boost your chances of conceiving, have intercourse from the ninth day of your cycle until three days after your basal body temperature rises. Unfortunately, not all women demonstrate these classic temperature patterns, so the basal body temperature method will not work for everyone.

- Cervical mucus method (aka the Billings method). Changes in hormones also cause changes in the thickness, amount, texture, and appearance of your cervical mucus throughout each cycle. By noting those changes over several cycles, you can predict ovulation.

How to Track Cervical Mucus

Every day, insert a finger into your vagina to collect cervical mucus and note the amount, color, and thickness or thinness. Place a drop between your index finger and thumb, and then spread your fingers to test the "stretchability" of the mucus—how long it stretches before breaking. After menstruation, cervical mucus is scant, thin, whitish to yellow, and only slightly sticky.

Just before ovulation, cervical mucus thickens, increases in amount, becomes clear and slippery—almost like uncooked egg white—and stretches over an inch before breaking.

Since these three natural methods for determining fertility are not 100 percent foolproof, your best bet is a combination of all three. You can also opt for a home kit, such as Ovuquick or Clearblue, that will tell you when you're ovulating by monitoring the presence and levels of LH, or a kit such as ClearPlan Easy Fertility Monitor, that measures estrogen metabolites plus LH levels in your urine. Be sure to follow the kit's directions carefully for accurate test results.

TREATING OVULATION DYSFUNCTIONS

One great advantage to boosting fertility with TCM is its reliance on "natural" methods—acupuncture, herbs, nutrition, meditation, and other lifestyle modifications—rather than on prescription drugs that can have harmful or uncomfortable side effects. In general, conventional medicine treats all ovulation dysfunctions in escalating stages:

- Progesterone supplementation. This type of hormone supplementation is used in women with luteal phase deficiencies.

- Ovulation induction agents. Another first treatment option in cases of women with highly irregular, anovulatory (not ovulating) cycles, is ovulation-inducing drugs. Clomiphene citrate, under such brand names as Clomid or Serophene, is the drug most often used to induce ovulation. In cases of luteal phase deficiency, ovulation-inducing drugs can at times be an alternative to progesterone supplementation. They are also sometimes used when infertility is unexplained, to give the ovaries a little jump start. Women using these drugs for ovulation problems typically use clomiphene citrate from day five to day nine of their cycle. This drug causes ovulation in about three-quarters of young, anovulatory women who take it, but only 35 to 40 percent actually become pregnant and carry a baby to term within a year.

The success rates of clomiphene citrate and acupuncture are therefore almost comparable, but clomiphene citrate and similar drugs can cause mood swings and other unpleasant side effects in a number of women. Being an antiestrogen, drugs such as clomiphene citrate can also cause a thinning of the uterine lining. It's pointless to take clomiphene citrate for more than six ovulatory cycles, since 95 percent of pregnancies on clomiphene citrate occur in the first six cycles and returns diminish after that. If you have poor cervical mucus or your partner's semen analysis is abnormal, in addition to your other ovulation issues, a conventional fertility doctor may recommend intrauterine insemination in combination with clomiphene citrate to bypass the poor mucus.

- Gonadotropins aka follicle-stimulating hormones (FSH) and luteinizing hormone (LH). If clomiphene citrate and similar drugs don't work, your doctor may next suggest gonadotropin medications such as Gonal-f, Follistim, or Repronex. These drugs stimulate the development of ovarian follicles and should always be closely monitored to make sure they don't hyperstimulate the ovaries. They are also commonly used in combination with intrauterine insemination. Women who use "fertility drugs" to stimulate ovulation may give birth to more than one baby because these drugs cause the ovaries to release multiple eggs instead of a single one.

• GnRH agonists. Lupron Depot is the most commonly used drug of this class, and it is a prime example of how doctors often employ a drug for its "off label" actions. "Off label" means the drug has not been FDA approved for the particular use. Lupron Depot, and other drugs in this class, can help infertility by suppressing the ability of the pituitary gland to stimulate the ovary at the wrong time. Evidence suggests that Lupron Depot increases pregnancy rates in IVF cycles because it is used to prevent ovulation from taking place before eggs can be retrieved from the ovaries. A brief course of Lupron Depot is followed by ovary-stimulating drugs that cause a rapid increase in estrogen level.

Side effects from these drugs may include such symptoms as hot flashes, bloating, mid-cycle pain, breast tenderness, nausea, dizziness, headaches, depression, anxiety, insomnia, and tiredness.

If you are unable to produce eggs due to poor ovarian function, conventional medicine also offers the possibility of egg donation to help you get pregnant. Eggs, donated by a young woman, are fertilized by your partner's sperm and then implanted in your uterus using in vitro fertilization and similar procedures that we describe in detail in chapter 7.

All these procedures are expensive and can produce mild to severe side effects, and there is controversy over possible long-term safety problems that we discuss in chapter 7. For these reasons, more and more people are opting for less-invasive, more-natural treatments such as TCM. In our clinic, we treat a variety of ovulation issues, as well as cervical mucus problems, with acupuncture and other TCM healing strategies with or without concomitant conventional medications and assisting techniques.

YOUR PARTNER'S NONSURGICAL PROBLEMS

In the last chapter we covered male infertility problems caused by such structural issues as varicoceles, obstructions in the epididymis, blockages or malformations of the ejaculatory ducts and the opening of the urethra. For all these problems, except mild forms of varicoceles, surgery is the answer.

However, when sperm cannot be delivered high enough into the vagina because of impotence, premature ejaculation, retrograde ejaculation and other ejaculatory dysfunctions, or hypospadias or epispadias, surgery may not have to be an option.

One major way conventional medicine resolves these problems is through artificial insemination (AI). With AI procedures, sperm is introduced into the female reproductive tract in ways other than sexual intercourse. Depending on the particular condition, this can be done through a number of different sperm preparation techniques, but generally it involves:

- Intra-cervical insemination through the cervix, in which case freshly ejaculated sperm is used.
- Intrauterine insemination in which sperm is "washed" to remove some undesirable component in the semen such as prostaglandins and to improve the sperms' function, then it is introduced into the uterine cavity

Prescription drugs are another conventional medical option that may partially correct such conditions as impotence, retrograde ejaculation, infections of the prostate or seminal vesicle, and even low sperm count.

Other, more rare types of nonsurgical conditions are treated by conventional medicine with hormone therapy, which attempts to boost levels of hormones in which the man is deficient or as a strategy to counter overly high levels of other hormones. Hormone therapy is an option for treating the following:

- Hypogonadotropic hypogonadism, also known as Kallmann syndrome, which is a rare and inherited disorder more common in males in which low levels of the hormones FSH and LH cause sex cells to function improperly. It is often accompanied by loss of the sense of smell, impaired hormone production, and failure of the testicles to produce sperm properly.
- Congenital adrenal hyperplasia, a group of disorders in which an enzyme necessary to produce certain male hormones is missing. The adrenal glands are not able to produce adequate amounts of steroid hormones called corticosteroids, two of which, glucocorticoids and mineralocorticoids, are active in the body. This causes blood levels of the hormones cortisol and aldosterone to lower, so the pituitary compensates by manufacturing overly high amounts of ACTH (adrenocorticotropic hormone), which, in turn, stimulates the adrenal cortex to produce more androgens (male steroid hormones) that lower fertility.
- Hyperprolactinemia, a condition in which blood levels of prolactin are too high. The pituitary gland produces

prolactin, a hormone that is abundant in pregnant and nursing women because it maintains milk production. However, nonpregnant women and men also have prolactin in their bloodstreams, and these levels vary throughout the day and night. Stress, medications, and tumors of the pituitary gland can cause an increase in prolactin production, and in men this condition can cause lack of libido and impotence. Treatment options depend on the underlying cause.

TCM AND HORMONE-RELATED INFERTILITY

Again, scientific research continues to add to the lengthy list of ailments that respond to acupuncture and other elements of TCM and many hormone imbalance–related fertility issues in women and men can be treated successfully with this age-old healing system.

The treatment of hormone imbalance–related fertility issues is where alternative modalities and conventional medicine can either complement each other or part ways. It's important to note that even conventional doctors are not in total agreement on several key fertility issues and how to treat them. For example, a study in Canada called ENDOCAN showed that patients with stage one and stage two endometriosis had significantly greater pregnancy rates once the condition was treated. However, a subsequent study conducted in Italy failed to show the same results.

Another controversy concerns luteal phase deficiency or defect. If tests find an excess of progesterone in the uterine lining, it's often assumed it will be difficult to sustain a pregnancy, and so estrogen injections are often prescribed to correct that imbalance. Yet American doctors A. C. Wentz and Georgeanna Jones, recognized authorities on the subject, recently recanted their original study conclusions, in which they claimed that luteal phase defect impairs fertility.

In general, conventional medicine approaches hormonal issues by attempting to adjust hormonal levels and stimulate endocrine function in order to restore the level of hormone balance that allows ovulation, egg fertilization, and implantation to take place.

TCM and other alternative and complementary physicians are keenly aware that hormonal imbalance can be caused by microscopically tiny changes in the endocrine system as well as any other dysfunctions in the entire mind-body complex. Two pitfalls of the conventional medical approach that prescribes hormones and hormone-stimulating drugs are, one, that these strategies do not address the underlying cause of the hormonal imbalance and therefore may not correct it. And, two, the hormone system can be thrown off by such minute excesses or deficiencies that drugs and supplements may not be capable of restoring hormonal balance with sufficient accuracy or for more than a brief period of time.

In my practice, we try to avoid these pitfalls by taking a broader, more inclusive view of the person rather than focusing exclusively on the body functions that appear to relate exclusively to fertility. Within the point of view shared by modern alternative medicine and traditional Asian healing practices, each patient is a unique entity composed of the interconnected matrix of body, mind, emotions, and spirit. This means that even if a fertility problem originates in an emotional, mental, or spiritual conflict, it can be effectively treated through the physical body or the mind, and vice versa. This holistic view also implies that your entire being should be addressed when dealing with any health problem, including infertility.

According to the holistic view, fertility problems can be lifestyle related, contributed to or the result of, for example, poor diet, lack of exercise or overexercise, and chronic stress. We in the West have developed a remarkable array of medical innovations to assist reproduction. Yet along with these advanced fertility technologies, we are also becoming increasingly subject to relentless performance pressure. Ironically, the anxiety created by this goal-oriented approach to reproduction can actually impede your ability to have a child. When worrying reaches obsessive levels, you lose your ability to let go and immerse yourself completely in a natural and spontaneous lovemaking experience. You are no longer an involved participant; you "go outside" to become a distanced observer who anxiously hopes that each time will finally be the time you become pregnant. After a series of "failed" attempts, the phenomenon becomes self-perpetuating, as your anxiety continues to build, taking you further and further from your goal of a successful pregnancy.

Nothing dampens sexual desire more than extreme self-consciousness and worry, and studies have shown that being relaxed, comfortable, and spontaneous when making love actually increases your chances of becoming pregnant.

Within this perspective, relaxing and letting go helps restore the energy flow and balance and therefore can dramatically increase your chances of conceiving and bearing a child—sometimes even more effectively than a course of hormones or drugs. Balanced hormone function also depends on sound general health and energy levels, good nutrition, the right type of exercise—or better yet, *activity*—and getting enough rest. You may also need to take supplements and herbs, especially if you are over thirty and your supply of essential hormones, proteins, antioxidants, and other substances has begun to dwindle. This is also a good time to explore traditional Eastern solutions—acupuncture, acupressure, yoga, and Taoist exercises—for strengthening and healing your reproductive organs and glands. These powerfully effective strategies that prevent and reverse fertility problems will be covered in detail in chapter 10.

If we are treating a patient for whom any fertility obstacles requiring a surgeon or medical doctor's attention have been ruled out, and she's eliminated tobacco or recreational drugs and excess alcohol, our next step to restoring fertility-boosting balance is to examine her health lifestyle in greater depth, including diet, exercise habits, stress load, and other environmental factors.

Again, all alternative and complementary approaches, including TCM, always begin with building a bigger picture of the patient's overall condition and health through a range of diagnostic strategies and tools, including, for example, TCM pulse diagnosis, in order to get at the root cause(s) of the imbalance(s) causing the hormone problem, which may not even be located in the sex organs or glands. As you will learn in chapter 11, even mental stress, particularly if it's constant and ongoing, can be enough to create a hormonal imbalance that suppresses ovulation and impairs fertility.

UNEXPLAINED INFERTILITY

Many couples who do not show abnormalities in infertility testing and/or have previously had a child become perplexed and frustrated when they don't conceive. You should know that just because you've been fertile in the past, that doesn't mean you are still fertile. In addition, unexplained infertility is also referred to as being sub-fertile, meaning you're just taking a long time to conceive, and all you really need for a successful pregnancy is a bit more patience. Although unexplained infertility can be frustrating, it may reassure you to know that it is quite prevalent and you are not alone. In fact, unexplained infertility occurs in 10 to 15 percent of all those who seek fertility help. Studies show that with appropriate treatment many patients with unexplained infertility will eventually conceive. In conventional medicine, the same strategies used to correct hormonal problems—ovulation-stimulating drugs and hormone supplementation—are employed for unexplained or sub-fertility problems in an attempt to shorten the amount of time it takes to conceive.

Our clinic results with unexplained infertility are excellent. This diagnosis responds reasonably well to TCM, because a TCM practitioner builds such a comprehensive diagnostic picture, including possible infertility factors a conventional physician would not even consider since they do not *seem* related to reproductive function. In addition, your treatment and diagnosis change each time you visit your TCM practitioner according to how you respond to the healing program that's been designed for you.

If you have unexplained infertility and have decided to take the conventional medical route, be sure to follow these steps:

- First make sure evaluation has been completed and you've had a laparoscopy to rule out endometriosis and other obstructions.

- Try gonadotropin therapy plus IUI.
- If that therapy doesn't work, then go to IVF.

IMMUNE PROBLEMS AND UNEXPLAINED INFERTILITY

In recent years, the role of the immune system in fertility—from conception through every stage of a pregnancy—has received increasing attention within conventional medical circles, a welcome sign that Western medicine is beginning to take a more holistic approach to healing. Within the conventional approach, the immune system is seen as the body's first line of defense. It recognizes foreign substances, such as cold viruses, that don't belong in the body, then attacks and destroys them. The immune system is made up of special proteins called antibodies that attach themselves to foreign substances and allow other immune cells to attack them. These other immune cells include special white blood cells produced by the lymph system that runs throughout the body. This is why you get swollen lymph glands when you are fighting off an infection. Other chemicals and proteins in the immune system also help fight and kill bacteria, viruses, and other foreign invaders. When your immune system is working at its peak, you are able to beat off infections.

In cases of unexplained infertility or repeated miscarriages, a conventional physician should consider testing you for antiphospholipid, antinuclear, antithyroid, and anti-sperm antibodies, as well as perform general tests to evaluate immune system function overall.

Immune System Disorders: The Western Point of View

These are some diagnoses given for immune system disorders that affect fertility:

Anti-phospholipid antibody syndrome, a lupuslike syndrome, can be present even in women without immune system disorders. This syndrome shows up in blood tests as positive markers called lupus anticoagulant and anti-cardiolipin antibodies, and it is believed to cause thickening of the blood (which reduces nutrient flow to your ovaries and uterine lining), difficulty in conceiving, risk of pregnancy loss, and, less commonly, fetal death or stillbirth in later pregnancies. Signs that you may have this syndrome include a history of blood clots, infertility, and recurrent miscarriages. If tests show you have those antibodies, you may have to be treated with anticoagulants (such as heparin, and/or baby aspirin) to enhance your fertility.

If you have suffered repeated miscarriages, the chances that it's due to this syndrome range from 5 to 10 percent. If you have lupus, the risk of miscarriage increases to 30 to 40 percent. If you have this syndrome and become pregnant, your pregnancy will need to be closely monitored with prenatal visits every one to two weeks up to delivery and frequent ultrasounds to make sure the fetus is thriving. You will also be advised about lifestyle changes to help the fetus develop safely.

Antinuclear antibodies (ANA) levels are measured by an antinuclear antibody test to discover the presence and amount of abnormal antibodies that attack the body's own tissues instead of performing the normal antibody function—defending the body from viruses, bacteria, and other foreign substances. The results of an ANA test are expressed in titres. A titre is a measure of how much the blood sample can be diluted before the presence of antibodies can no longer be detected. A titre of one to eighty (1:80) means that antibodies could be last detected when one part of the blood sample was diluted by eighty parts of another liquid (usually a dilute salt solution). The larger the second number, the more antibodies that are present. We all have a small amount of these antibodies, but about 5 percent of the general population has a larger number than normal, and about half of these people suffer as a result from autoimmune diseases such as systemic lupus erythematosus or rheumatoid arthritis. These autoimmune diseases must be diagnosed through other, more specific tests that measure specific titres present for each disease. The presence of an elevated ANA titer can suggest a more subtle syndrome similar to the presence of anti-phospholipid antibodies, and a doctor may consider giving you some form of anticoagulation treatment.

Certain factors, including specific medications and aging, can give a false high ANA. Steroids, however, can produce a false low result.

Antithyroid antibodies create problems with the thyroid gland. A doctor diagnoses overactive thyroid (hyperthyroidism) or underactive thyroid (hypothyroidism) through blood tests that measure hormones secreted by the thyroid and also TSH, the thyroid-stimulating hormone secreted by the pituitary. Simply put, hyperthyroidism speeds your metabolism up, while hypothyroidism slows it down. In hyperthyroidism, you have low levels of TSH, while in hypothyroidism, you have higher TSH levels, as your pituitary gland is producing more in an attempt to get your thyroid going.

Hypothyroidism can cause weight gain, difficulty in losing weight, dry skin and hair, fatigue, hoarseness, muscle cramps, depression, high cholesterol, mild hypertension, and inability to tolerate the cold.

Hyperthyroidism can affect bowel habits, cause weight loss, hand tremors, increased perspiration, irritability, trouble sleeping, weakness in the upper arms and thighs, cardiac arrhythmia, infertility, and thinning bones.

Most cases of hypothyroidism result from an autoimmunity dysfunction. The best estimates are that hypothyroidism, much more common in women than men, affects one woman in eleven. In our experience, hypothyroidism occurs far more often in women who have difficulties conceiving than in fertile women and is the single most common physical abnormality in our female infertility patients. Not always detected, it is perhaps the most common endocrine/immunologic cause of female infertility—sometimes a patient can be clinically hypothyroid and all her blood test results are normal. A trial thyroid supplementation is not conventionally offered, but from an alternative medical perspective, it should be considered.

The thyroid gland is located in the center of the neck, near the larynx (voice box), and it secretes hormones that control metabolism, as well as impacts on your menstrual cycle and ability to conceive. Endocrinologists estimate that approximately 14 million people in the United States have some type of thyroid disease, but at least half remain undiagnosed.

The Colorado Thyroid Disease Prevalence Study acknowledges that thyroid dysfunction is widely underdiagnosed by the conventional blood tests that check blood hormone levels to determine if a patient has hypothyroidism (underactive thyroid) or hyperthyroidism (overactive thyroid). The study also found that 40 percent of the subjects who were taking thyroid medications still had abnormal levels of TSH, an indicator of continuing thyroid dysfunction.

One reason for the large numbers of undiagnosed thyroid problems today is that levels of the thyroid-stimulating hormone secreted by the pituitary gland can appear to be within normal levels on conventional blood tests, but you can suffer nevertheless from symptoms of underactive thyroid, including impaired fertility. Slightly low thyroid levels can worsen over time, so even a slight deviation from the norm should be taken seriously, especially when infertility is an issue. Determining whether problems such as high cholesterol, hoarseness, fatigue, or infertility are related to a thyroid disorder can require a bit of medical detective work, since each of these symptoms can be related to entirely different conditions.

Even when thyroid disease is diagnosed, experts are divided on whether or not to treat these slight deviations from the norm, although some doctors believe that a trial course of therapeutic medication is justified to see if a particular dose level relieves symptoms. In the case of thyroid-related immune disorders, which are more likely to grow more serious over time, starting medication before the disease progresses is considered a good option.

A simple way to check your own thyroid function is a temperature test that can detect potential metabolic disturbances that conventional tests can miss. The test is performed by you, then interpreted by your doctor. All you have to do is take your body temperature upon waking by placing a thermometer (not digital) under your armpit, for three days in a row, beginning on the third day of your menstrual cycle. If your body temperature consistently registers less than 97.5°F, a trial of thyroid medication may be in order.

While thyroid problems are not diagnosed as such by TCM practitioners, they may be corrected, in part, as the goal of restoring overall energetic balance is reached through natural means—acupuncture as well as nutritional, herbal, and lifestyle strategies.

Anti-sperm antibodies can be produced by you or your partner. They may affect the reproductive process by interfering with sperm survival and motility, as well as sperm's ability to pass through your cervical mucus. Clearly these antibodies may impair fertilization and it is little wonder that scientists are trying to develop a contraceptive vaccine that utilizes them to prevent pregnancy. Despite all the hurdles put up by anti-sperm antibodies, however, you can become pregnant with assisted reproductive techniques using sperm washing to remove antibodies if they are present in the semen. These antibodies are detected in the blood, cervical mucus, and seminal fluid by antibody tests. The definitive treatment for anti-sperm antibodies in the male is intracytoplasmic sperm injections (ICSI) with IVF, although TCM herbs have also been shown in trials to help treat them.

A conventional physician can check for any allergic reaction you may have by obtaining your blood and vaginal secretions at mid-cycle, when you're ovulating. This means you should be monitoring your cycle and cervical mucus by the methods described earlier in this chapter. If you choose to use an LH detection home kit, do the urine test in the mid to late morning, before you've taken in any liquids that could distort results. If all indications are that you are ovulating, see your doctor so he or she can collect blood and vaginal secretion samples the next day. Avoid douching (a bad idea at any time) within twenty-four hours before collecting vaginal secretion samples.

Immune factors and fertility remains a controversial subject among fertility specialists, especially since the same fertility treatments will be prescribed for unexplained infertility whether or not any antibodies are present to suggest autoimmune problems. Also, it's not possible to tell when early miscarriage results from failure of the embryo to implant or from unexplained infertility. Some experts even theorize that sperm antibodies found either in you or your partner may have no effect on your fertility at all. This supports some experts' contention that widespread use of immune testing in fertility practices may not be warranted, because no direct cause and effect has been conclusively determined between immune issues and reproductive failure. In addition, some medical experts even charge that the therapies employed when immune factors have been diagnosed can cause harm.

ALTERNATIVE APPROACHES TO IMMUNE PROBLEMS AND UNEXPLAINED INFERTILITY

As you now realize, TCM practitioners consider true healing to result from addressing underlying cause(s) of illness and dysfunction—as opposed to focusing on suppressing symptoms—and then by boosting the body's innate self-correcting healing mechanisms through acupuncture, herbs, nutritional and lifestyle modifications, meditation, and other strategies. Practitioner and patient work as partners because much of any healing process involves heightening your awareness of the workings of your mind-body system and modifying your lifestyle. Autoimmune disorders are a particular challenge because they can be controlled but are not easily cured—by either Western or Eastern medicine. Yet because TCM is so safe and works on such a deep level to protect and restore health, this natural and holistic modality can be your best option for immune system disorders that cause infertility.

In 1995, a team from Shanghai Medical University reported on the use of an ancient Chinese herbal formula called Zhibai Dihuang to treat the infertile couples with anti-sperm antibodies in their blood. It was found that the antibodies were converted to negative in 81.3 percent of couples after treatment, and eight successful pregnancies resulted within nine months after the antibodies' conversion. The negative status was maintained throughout the course of all the pregnancies.

Because a complementary physician considers not just the whole person—body and mind—but also that person within his or her world, this approach is particularly helpful in showing you how to avoid the estrogenic toxic chemicals that seem to be present everywhere we turn, especially in our own homes.

In an age of medical specialization, where body functions are parsed and turned over to the care of experts, many of us sense that we have lost a necessary holistic view of treating the person, not only as a complex and individual entity, but also as an integral part of the natural world. No wonder you and so many others who are trying to get pregnant find yourselves turning back the clock, seeking out traditional healing systems such as TCM, or blending this age-old practice with modern medical science for a complementary approach.

Before we discuss how you can combine TCM with the array of cutting-edge fertility techniques offered by modern medical science, let's take a look in the next chapter at ART, assisted reproductive technologies.

Chapter 7

The Art of ART: Assisted Reproductive Technologies

Intrauterine insemination, intra-cervical insemination, in vitro fertilization, preimplantation genetic diagnosis, introcytoplasmic sperm injection, gamete intrafallopian transfer, zygote intrafallopian transfer, frozen embryo transfer, donor eggs—these are the daunting names of the cutting-edge fertility treatments grouped together as assisted reproductive technologies (ART), the best modern Western medical science has to offer. Modern medicine has created brand-new opportunities for the fertility challenged.

ART treatments themselves can be formidable—expensive, time-consuming, uncomfortable, and not always successful—and this may be a step you are not prepared to take. Nonetheless, in our practice we've experienced great success combining TCM treatments with ART treatments given by fertility specialists, particularly in cases when fertility issues with the man or woman make conception through sexual intercourse unlikely.

You will learn more about the nutritional, herbal, and lifestyle aspects of TCM and our clinic programs in chapters 8 through 11. In this chapter, we will briefly guide you through various procedures grouped together as ART, in case one of them becomes your option.

INTRAUTERINE INSEMINATION (IUI)

For an IUI procedure, the man gives a sperm sample and the laboratory separates sperm from semen in order to prepare the sperm in a special culture medium. The lab also should separate more motile sperm from less active ones. The sperm can be frozen for later use or injected when fresh into the uterus via a catheter (a thin rubber tube) at the time of ovulation. IUI is often performed in conjunction with fertility drugs such as clomiphene citrate, Repronex, Gonal-f, or Follistim. Of course, there's no guarantee that the sperm will fertilize an egg or even that an egg will make it to the fallopian tube to be fertilized. IUI is indicated for mild sperm problems, cervical factors, or unexplained infertility. The cost for IUI is much lower than those of most other ART procedures—and the chances of success per attempt range from 10 percent (with clomiphene citrate) to 25 percent (with gonadotropins) in young couples.

INTRA-CERVICAL INSEMINATION (ICI)

In this relatively simple procedure that takes about five minutes, the doctor inserts a speculum into the vagina and then places semen into the cervix with a plastic catheter. Sometimes a sponge or cap is placed into the vagina for about six hours, before removing the speculum, in order to keep the sperm from leaking out. ICI is generally less effective and is medically indicated in couples who are young and have sexual or intercourse related problems.

IN VITRO FERTILIZATION (IVF)

In this procedure, mature eggs are taken from the ovaries and then fertilized with sperm in the laboratory. Before the eggs can be retrieved for any ART procedure, a woman must undergo daily injections of gonadotropins for about two weeks up to ovulation at the mid-point of her cycle. These drugs stimulate the ovaries to recruit multiple eggs instead of just one and stimulate those eggs to maturity. The woman's blood estrogen levels will be closely monitored, and ultrasound will check if eggs are maturing in the follicles. Her drug dose may be adjusted according to her response. An injection called human chorionic gonadotropin (HCG) will be given to further mature the eggs. Thirty-four to thirty-six hours after HCG, the eggs will be retrieved from the follicles using needle aspiration guided by vaginal ultrasound.

The number of eggs retrieved can vary greatly from woman to woman; however, the average number of eggs retrieved in women under the age of thirty-five is about ten to twelve per retrieval. The eggs are not necessarily gathered from every follicle seen on the ultrasound, as most women need to have fifteen to twenty follicles of varying sizes in order for ten to twelve eggs to be collected. Also, not all the eggs will be mature; some will be too mature and some too premature.

For fertilization, eggs are usually placed with sperm on a petri dish and incubated overnight. The next day, they will be checked for fertilization. In couples whose sperm are suboptimal, intracytoplasmic sperm injection (ICSI) will be done. A microscope guides a glass instrument called a pipette that holds the egg in place while another pipette holding a single sperm will inject the sperm into the egg. After these eggs are cultured overnight, they are checked again for evidence of fertilization. Those that have been fertilized are incubated for three to five days before they are transferred back to the uterus; at three days, they are pre-embryos, and at five days, they are blastocysts. Two to four, depending on the woman's age, are placed in the uterus using a catheter inserted through the cervix. The remaining viable embryos may be frozen for future attempts.

The average cost per IVF attempt ranges from $10,000 to $15,000, and the odds of success per attempt depend on the female's age and the particular IVF program.

No one can say for sure why, in some cases, IVF doesn't work. In part, it has to do with the individual patient's case. To assess ovarian reserve, one can test cycle day three FSH and estradiol hormonal levels. It's important to take an ultrasound to evaluate the number of "resting" follicles in both ovaries. In some patients, a clomiphene challenge test is recommended. Again, the doctor should have checked the uterine cavity to make sure it's normal before embarking on IVF.

Be careful to use what you are learning in this book to ensure that all the other diagnostic tests are always performed before attempting IVF.

On the other hand, in some cases, it's only after IVF fails that other reasons why pregnancy isn't taking place become apparent. These reasons include abnormal egg quality, abnormal fertilization, or abnormal embryo development in cases when a normal-looking embryo has functional deficiencies.

Embryo transfer is usually done three days after eggs have been retrieved and fertilized, when a normal embryo has between six and ten cells. Five days after the eggs have been retrieved, when the embryo has become a blastocyst, it begins to expand as the cells differentiate. This is the embryonic stage at which a fertilized embryo would normally leave the fallopian tube and reach the uterus. So some experts believe five days after the egg has been retrieved and fertilized is the optimal time to implant the embryo, as it more closely follows the course of nature. While studies show that pregnancy rates are similar between patients whose eggs were transferred at three and five days, only two or fewer embryos are needed for a successful pregnancy if transfer is done at five days, thereby decreasing the possibility of a risky multiple pregnancy. On the other hand, the embryo quality can be compromised after three days in the lab, which means that the ability of the lab to protect the egg is crucial. In addition, only 50 percent of embryos make it to the blastocyst stage, suggesting that natural selection is at work, eliminating some embryos in order to ensure genetic normalcy.

IVF success rates have improved dramatically in the last decade and can be used to treat most conditions that cause infertility. Two major problems IVF does not treat well, however, are significant uterine problems that cannot be repaired surgically and advanced age of a woman (over forty years old). Some small studies suggest another possible problem can lower the chance for success with IVF—endometriosis, especially for women who have undergone surgery to remove endometriosis from the ovaries, which invariably compromises ovarian reserve. This could cause a poor response to ovary-stimulating drugs, leading to fewer eggs retrieved and fewer embryos formed. Surgery to remove endometriosis from the ovaries also can reduce blood supply to the ovary, which lowers response to ovary-stimulating drugs. However, women who have had their endometriosis treated by surgery and who do respond to ovary-stimulating drugs have the same chance of a successful pregnancy as women with no history of endometriosis.

IVF and Uterine Problems

Even if a woman conceives through IVF, the live birthrate for women with an unicornuate uterus (a condition in which only half the uterus has developed normally), is likely to be reduced dramatically because of a high chance of miscarriage in the second trimester or premature delivery. However, excellent obstetrical care and a lot of bed rest can put the chances for a successful pregnancy at 15 to 30 percent.

IVF and Age

If you are older than forty, you should know that the natural reduction in fertility that occurs over time increases dramatically around age forty. For most women age forty-four, the chance that a single cycle of IVF will result in a live birth is well under 5 percent. Therefore, IVF is rarely performed in women over forty-four years old, because its chances for success are so low.

PREIMPLANTATION GENETIC DIAGNOSIS (PGD)

If you've suffered from repeated miscarriages, IVF may not solve your problem. A particular type of genetic counseling called preimplantation genetic diagnosis (PGD) in combination with IVF could be the answer, as some women are predisposed to a high number of genetically abnormal embryos. More and more clinics are relying on PGD, which can offer aneuploidy screening for women who've undergone recurrent miscarriages despite otherwise normal evaluations. Aneuploidy screening allows doctors to evaluate a percentage of chromosomes in order to determine whether or not an embryo is normal. Evidence suggests that incidence of genetically abnormal embryos increases sharply with women over thirty-seven. However, women who produce low numbers of embryos through IVF do not benefit from the selection process afforded by PGD, because this type of screening involves biopsy of the embryo, which means there's risk of impact on the growth of the embryos.

INTRACYTOPLASMIC SPERM INJECTION (ICSI)

ICSI is an advanced reproductive technology used to enhance the fertilization phase of IVF in the case of sperm-related infertility. A single sperm is injected into a mature egg, and the fertilized egg is then placed either in the uterus or a fallopian tube. If the sperm cannot be collected through masturbation because of a blockage, they are surgically removed through the scrotum. Men with very little or no sperm in their semen can undergo surgical procedures on the sperm tubes or testicles to remove sperm for ICSI. Men in this category should be fully evaluated by a urologist, which includes undergoing genetic counseling before attempting ICSI or IVF. ICSI costs in the range of $10,000 and has a 50 percent success rate.

GAMETE INTRAFALLOPIAN TRANSFER (GIFT)

In this procedure, eggs and sperm are placed in a fallopian tube through a laparoscopy. The procedure, however, has become obsolete as IVF laboratory procedures have improved. It is also unsuitable if tubal or sperm problems are involved.

ZYGOTE INTRAFALLOPIAN TRANSFER (ZIFT)

For ZIFT, sperm fertilize eggs in the lab, and those eggs that have been successfully fertilized are placed in a fallopian tube via laparoscopy on the day after egg retrieval. Again, the technique is no longer practical as it cannot offer any information on embryo development and it is unsuitable in women with tubal problems.

FROZEN EMBRYO TRANSFER (FET)

This procedure uses surplus embryos from previous IVF cycles that were frozen and stored for possible implantation in the uterus at a future date. The success rate is 50 to 67 percent that of a fresh cycle. Some couples with successful results even opt to donate their embryos to other couples that cannot use their own sperm and eggs.

DONOR EGGS

This procedure uses a donor woman's eggs, which are then fertilized with the male partner's sperm and transferred to the infertile woman's uterus. Egg donation can be performed anonymously or the egg donor can be known to the recipent couple. If egg donors are young (typically they are under thirty), success rates can approach 60 to 70 percent per attempt.

MAKING CHOICES

Hopefully, you won't need to invest the considerable money, time, and trouble ART requires, but if your options do come down to ART, you can take comfort in knowing that you are fortunate to live in a time when this level of fertility assistance is possible.

Keep in mind, however, that success rates for ART are not overwhelming. In addition, approximately 25 percent of all live births resulting from ART may be multiple births (twins, triplets, or higher-order multiples) as compared to 2 percent in natural pregnancies. Although infertile couples may welcome the idea of multiple births, multiple pregnancies are riskier than singleton or twin pregnancies and sometimes pose an ethical and emotional dilemma when one or more embryos need to be selectively terminated because of overcrowding in the uterus.

Another key consideration before embarking on ART is to make sure your fertility specialist has evaluated even the less obvious factors in your situation so you have more therapeutic choices. Let's say, for example, you chose the conventional route and underwent drug therapy to stimulate your ovaries.

You produced four good-quality eggs that were then fertilized and implanted in your uterus. If your uterine lining wasn't checked for thickness, those embryos may not implant if the lining is too thin. This is a complicated issue, because your endometrial thickness can be measured by ultrasound, but, sometimes, even a lining with normal thickness may not be adequate. You could compare it to trying to plant flowers in your garden. You measured out the right amount of topsoil, but if the soil quality is poor or poorly irrigated, the flowers may not grow, despite what seemed to be an adequate layer of soil. Generally, the endometrium is considered adequate at 7 or 8 mm in thickness, but some women have delivered a healthy baby with an endometrium measuring less than 7 mm. The usual approach is to increase stimulation drugs during the next IVF attempt, so that the woman will have higher estradiol levels that should develop a thicker endometrium. If an endometrium does not develop to 7 or 8 mm in thickness, conventional medicine has no solution. This is an uncommon problem that affects only 2 to 3 percent of women. It's important to keep in mind that TCM not only improves ovulation and egg quality, it also helps improve the quality of the endometrial lining in preparation for nurturing a developing fetus. Alternative methods such as baby aspirin and white willow bark that are used to increase pelvic blood flow may also enhance the quality of the uterine lining.

When choosing an ART program, you, your partner, and your doctor must take into account the expense, convenience, quality of care, and the program's track record. It's not unusual for some couples to spend as much as $50,000 per cycle on ART programs.

The stress of undergoing ART is another factor you should consider. When the stakes are so high—because your hopes and expenses are so high—you may find yourself on an emotional roller coaster. Because you are taking fertility drugs, as well as timing ovulation, intercourse, and implantation to the most advantageous times in your cycle, and then waiting at least two weeks to find out if you're pregnant, it's difficult to know whether your emotional instability is rooted in emotional or physical causes or both. In chapter 11, you'll learn easy, quick tips for reducing stress to increase your chances of becoming pregnant. For now, it's helpful just to know that it's normal to feel stressed out whenever you undergo such heroic procedures to become pregnant.

Again, before choosing an ART procedure, use the fertility education you're gaining here to ensure that you and your partner have been thoroughly evaluated so you are fully aware of your options and your time and money will not be wasted.

WHEN ENOUGH MAY BE ENOUGH

How do you decide enough is enough? Remember that the longer something has not happened, the less likely it will happen. A young couple who's just started trying to conceive has a 25 percent chance of pregnancy per each month of trying, but that figure drops to about 2 percent per month after two years. The same figures are true of IVF. The number of IVF cycles that you probably should consider undertaking is up to five or six, but the principle of diminishing returns still holds. This is because each cycle can yield important information about the quality of sperm, eggs, and embryo. If the first cycle shows that the quality of sperm, egg, or embryo is poor, a second cycle may or may not be recommended, as chances for success are low. However, if you have responded well to ovarian stimulation and embryo quality is good, then it could be reasonable to try a second cycle or more. These are highly personal decisions and you ought to discuss each cycle carefully and consider all angles when consulting with your fertility specialist. Let's say ovarian stimulation has been good enough to result in ten to twelve eggs on average in two cycles, so you are considered to have a normal response to ovarian stimulation. Yet you haven't become pregnant. In that case, your doctor might look to a problem with the sperm fertilizing the egg or some problem with the eggs themselves. Sperm problems frequently can be treated effectively with intracytoplasmic sperm injection. However, if ICSI is performed and a pregnancy still hasn't resulted, the reason could be a reduction in egg quality over the course of the IVF cycles, although another cause could be widespread but subtle sperm defects that do not reveal themselves upon routine sperm testing or when undertaking ICSI. The decision to keep going would depend on the quality of the embryos and their development. If embryo development seems to be good, then it might be worth another try. However, if embryo development is not good or egg quality appears to be abnormal, the chances of a successful pregnancy through IVF would be low.

Again, it's always important to weigh the emotional and financial costs of IVF cycles against other options, including adoption. And remember, when you add acupuncture and alternative therapies to the IVF process, sperm and egg quality, fertilization, and implantation improve.

POSSIBLE RISKS OF FERTILITY DRUGS AND ART

The safety of fertility drugs and ART remains controversial. My personal belief is that ART is relatively safe. The following are the major points of contention regarding ART:

- Fertility drugs have a potential to cause cancer. There has been a question for some time about whether fertility drugs are connected with ovarian cancer. Suppressing ovulation with birth control pills appears to lower the risk of ovarian cancer, and since fertility drugs increase the number of ovulations, there is a theoretical reason why they might increase ovarian cancer risk. Most studies have not found an increased risk of ovarian cancer in women who have used fertility drugs.
- Fertility medications can cause ovarian hyperstimulation. The *ASRM Bulletin* acknowledges that this condition can be severe but states that this is a rare side effect that affects less than 1 percent of women who undergo ART. Long-term injury is even less common.
- IVF increases the risk of ectopic pregnancy. Since tubal disease is such a common indication for IVF, patients with this problem already have a high risk for ectopic pregnancy whether they conceive naturally or through IVF. In fact, notes the *ASRM Bulletin*, studies indicate that IVF actually reduces the risk of ectopic pregnancy.
- IVF is inappropriately recommended for patients with undiagnosed male infertility or abnormalities of the uterus. IVF is the standard conventional medical option for those with low sperm count or motility. How-

ever, before you embark on ART, uterine abnormalities should be ruled out. If your fertility specialist does not do this, find another doctor.

Let's conclude this discussion of the "art of ART" by reminding you that TCM generally produces no harmful side effects and that even if you do embark on the conventional route to a successful pregnancy, your odds of conceiving with ART will be enhanced if you combine those technologies with traditional Chinese medicine techniques such as acupuncture and other alternative methods.

Chapter 8

Boost Your Fertility with Hormone-Balancing Foods

If you want to become pregnant, you may already be aware that diet and nutrition count because you need to ready the "home" you will provide for an embryo to develop into a full-term infant. Yet you may not know exactly how important diet can be to fertility, or realize that providing yourself with the right nutrition could be the deciding factor in your getting pregnant.

First of all, depending on your particular condition, you may need to gain rather than lose weight. Just as people tend to believe that all exercise is healthy, most people believe that dieting to lose weight is generally a good idea. Yet, in certain situations—such as when you're trying to become pregnant—exercise and dieting can be harmful, especially if practiced to an extreme.

Exceptions to the rule that *not* dieting boosts your fertility include your having PCOS or that you are borderline diabetic with hyperinsulinism or so-called metabolic syndrome X. In these cases, overnourishment and overproduction of insulin and insulin-related hormones may be the root cause of your infertility, so dieting with increased physical activity and/or sugar-reducing drugs will enhance your fertility.

EATING MORE CAN FUEL YOUR FERTILITY

The study of evolution and Darwin's theory of the survival of the fittest tell us the species that thrive and survive are the ones best able to adapt to their specific environments. We know that human physiology is not fixed, and that an important survival tactic is the ability to make continual bodily adjustments in response to changes in the environment. Part of our human adaptation to a changing environment involves reproducing when food is plentiful enough to nourish an expectant mother and her infant, and not reproducing when nourishment is too scarce to support pregnancy and new life. This is an example of how your reproductive drive works in tandem with your built-in survival strategies. You can see, therefore, that dieting can be subconsciously interpreted to mean there's a lack of sufficient nutrition in your environment to support a pregnancy. Whenever you diet, your body gets a message that this is not a good time to reproduce, and your "fertilistat" level lowers.

So if you want to become pregnant, make sure you take in

sufficient nutrition. How much fat should you have in order to maximize your chances of a successful pregnancy? You must maintain a normal healthy body weight, using the body mass index (BMI) scale, or up to 5 to 10 percent in excess of that. To calculate your body mass index (which correlates weight to height, regardless of gender), multiply your weight in pounds by 703 and then divide that number by your height in inches squared. Or simply look up your ideal BMI in a reference book. The ideal BMI for a woman trying to conceive is twenty to twenty-seven. If you are on either side of that range, follow the advice you'll get in this chapter, and/or talk to your doctor about how to adjust your eating and/or exercise habits.

As you already know, it doesn't take too much to impair fertility. If your body fat falls too low (to a level below 15 percent), your body protects itself by greatly reducing estrogen production and stopping ovulation to conserve energy. So, if you are underweight, make sure you take in at least 30 percent of your daily calories from healthy and energy-concentrated fat sources such as olive oil, ocean fish, and others you'll learn about in this chapter.

Experts differ on exactly how overweight can affect fertility. One study found that the overweight women in a group of infertile patients taking ovary-stimulation drugs and undergoing intrauterine insemination had a higher chance of success than normal-weight women undergoing ovarian hyperstimulation with intrauterine insemination. On the other hand, another study of women undergoing artificial insemination procedures showed that obesity is associated with an impaired response to ovarian stimulation and increased risk of early pregnancy loss before six weeks' gestation. However, this study also indicated that underweight was not related to an impaired outcome of artificial insemination procedures.

Most studies connect obesity to infertility, and it's been demonstrated that polycystic ovary syndrome, which can impair ovulation, is linked to obesity. If you are seriously overweight, weight loss can enhance your fertility. But lose the weight *before* you try to get pregnant, because dieting at the same time you're trying to conceive may be counterproductive.

Estrogen is a wonderful hormone that allows for conception and pregnancy and keeps your skin smoothed and toned. But in excess, it can cause problems. Why do some of us have too much estrogen? Possible reasons include:

- excess weight
- chronic stress
- nutritional deficiencies
- environmental toxins
- estrogens in the food supply

SYMPTOMS OF ESTROGEN DOMINANCE

The following symptoms could indicate estrogen dominance:

- premenstrual syndrome
- irregular and/or painful menstrual periods
- lack of ovulation
- heavy periods
- breast tenderness
- fluid retention

Estrogen dominance and other hormonal imbalance conditions can lead to several problems, including blood sugar imbalances, endometriosis, fibroids, PMS, perhaps some female cancers, and, yes, infertility. Yet any hormonal imbalance can be corrected by taking a natural approach that includes the right foods in the right amounts along with acupuncture and, if needed, herbs and nutritional supplements and other lifestyle modifications. The right diet provides the quality nutrients the body needs in order to promote free energy flow so it can function in a balanced and efficient way, manufacture essential hormones at optimum levels, and release these natural chemicals into your bloodstream at precisely the right times.

Now, let's examine how hormone function is closely linked to the types of foods you eat, the quality of your food, and the ways in which your food is prepared, digested, and assimilated into your body.

The best fertility prescription for you may not be drugs but healthy eating, a common missing element in people's fertility plans. Follow the nutritional advice you are about to discover, and you will be taking an important step toward greater health, proper hormone balance, and a successful pregnancy.

It's all up to you.

HOW FOODS IMPACT FERTILITY

Simple Sugars and Refined Starches Simple sugars and refined starches deteriorate health and create the following negative effects:

- Hormone imbalance. That energy "rush" from a candy bar or glazed doughnut lasts all of fifteen minutes to half an hour. It comes from a sharp rise in your blood sugar levels, but that "high" soon switches direction and plummets downward, leaving you drained and exhausted. You drag through your days, feeling depleted, emotionally unstable, and constantly tired. Other possible symptoms of this blood sugar imbalance include daytime panic attacks and waking up in the middle of the night, sweating, heart racing. You are in a state of emergency because your adrenal glands are secreting extra cortisol—the so-called flight or fight hormone—in an attempt to replenish your system's sugar levels because sugar is essential fuel for every body system. Over time, too much cortisol stimulated by chronic low blood sugar levels weakens your adrenal glands to the point where they produce lower levels of sex hormones. This can lead to hormone imbalance that impacts fertility.

- B vitamin deficiency. Manufacturing excess cortisol eventually uses up nutrients needed for proper hormone balance and fertility. These include the B vitamins, especially B_6, and magnesium. Vitamin B deficiency may make you vulnerable to some harmful effects of stress, another fertility buster.
- Overly high insulin levels. In order to get all this sugar out of the blood and into cells, where it's converted into energy, the pancreas has to keep secreting insulin. Excess insulin secretion eventually causes insulin resistance, which is known to be associated with infertility.
- Compromised immune response. Some research shows that just a single teaspoon of sugar can reduce immunity for up to four hours.

Your best bet is to avoid sugar, including honey, altogether. Satisfy your sweet tooth with plenty of fruits. For example, treat yourself to a fruit smoothie blending fresh fruit and ice cubes. Maple syrup in small amounts is okay, especially in cooking. Stevia, a South American plant with even more concentrated sweetening power than sugar, does not affect your blood sugar levels.

Bad Fats All fats are not bad for fertility. In fact, certain fats protect fertility because they help absorb and store proper amounts of fat-soluble vitamins A, D, E, and K—all of which ensure reproductive health. Good fats also are the most concentrated source of body energy on the cellular level. Saturated fats, found mostly in red meat, dairy products, and shellfish, are bad fats. *"Hydrogenated"* or *"partially hydrogenated" oils* (aka *trans-fatty acids),* are even worse for you, because hydrogenated fats are chemically altered to become solid at room temperature, just like saturated fats. Margarine is a good example of a hydrogenated or partially hydrogenated fat. It was developed from a liquid fat and altered to become solid at room temperature so it could substitute for butter.

Eating these bad fats replaces healthy essential fats in the membranes of your body cells. Saturated fats contain an essential fatty acid called arachidonic acid that the body uses to produce inflammatory reactions and cramping. So if you suffer from the symptoms of fibroids, endometriosis, and other estrogen-dominant states, a diet heavy in meat and dairy products will aggravate, rather than reverse, those symptoms. Of course, all nonorganic meat and dairy products contain residues of antibiotics, hormones, insecticides, and pesticides that can also play havoc with your hormone system.

What to Use Instead of Bad Fats

Use only small amounts of cold-pressed, unrefined, polyunsaturated oils, such as canola and sesame, for cooking, or the monounsaturated oil—olive oil. Over the long term, these oils actually can help remove harmful plaque that builds up on blood vessel walls from a diet of saturated fats. Olive oil makes a healthy and tasty dressing for salads and other foods. Flaxseed oil is another oil that can be used as a salad dressing.

Coffee Drinking up to one or two cups of coffee daily probably does not hurt your fertility, according to a 2003 report from the Center for the Evaluation of Risks to Human Reproduction at the National Institutes of Health. But whether coffee (or caffeine) affects female fertility in larger amounts is debatable; one large modern study found that women who consumed 300 mg or more of caffeine a day took longer to conceive than those who consumed less or none. There is also clear evidence that 300 mg or more of caffeine a day can raise your risk of miscarriage. A study by researchers at Duke University Medical Center shows that caffeine taken in the morning amplifies stress consistently throughout the day. It may well be the amplified stress from coffee and caffeine that indirectly affects fertility, as stress and your mind play such important roles in reproduction. However, according to Brazilian researchers, in the case of men, coffee has been shown to enhance sperm function.

Try black or green tea. You may be asking, "How about caffeine in tea?" We suspect that any harm from coffee may not be from the caffeine but from other ingredients in the brew, as drinking tea, caffeinated or not, seems to be one of the more established dietary means to promote fertility. A study from the Kaiser Permanente Medical Care Program in Northern California shows that drinking half a cup or more of green or black tea daily can double your chances of conception. A Dutch study shows that three to four cups of tea a day can quadruple your chances of becoming pregnant per cycle. Scientists are now examining tea's chemical compounds to find out why. One leading theory is that antioxidant compounds in tea protect DNA from damage, thereby decreasing the number of unhealthy embryos. However, a tea-drinking habit may also be linked to a healthier lifestyle in general.

Alcohol Studies indicate some healthful benefits of red wine may help lower cholesterol and are good for the heart. However, women with fertility-impairing hormone imbalance conditions should avoid excessive alcohol because of its potential harmful effects on the body. And when alcohol is desired, always choose wine over liquor and beer, and red over white because of the rich presence of antioxidants in red wine.

Carbonated Sodas These are packed with sugar or artificial sweeteners, sometimes caffeine, and are high in phosphates, which interfere with calcium absorption. Caffeinated sodas stimulate the adrenal glands to produce more cortisol, the stress hormone, thereby aggravating anxiety and fatigue, and promoting hormone imbalance.

THE DIET TO FUEL FERTILITY

Now that we've talked about bad nutrition, let's explore further what you should eat to boost fertility. Before we get into traditional Chinese medicine's dietary recommendations, let's cover general good nutrition for women who want to get pregnant. Proteins, fats, and carbohydrates are present in all foods in various proportions, but it's important you get them in quality forms. This means good nutrition is a matter of selecting foods that are packed with quality versions of these three elements. We know this is important, because people who live in cultures where the diet includes quality nutrition—from fresh fruits, vegetables, nuts, seeds, soy products, grains, and fewer hydrogenated fats—experience far less incidence of infertility.

Although no single diet plan is perfect for everyone, most of us do well on a diet of high-quality foods that supply anywhere from 30 to 35 percent carbohydrates, 25 to 40 percent protein, and 20 to 30 percent fats.

Dr. Allan Warshowsky, a respected integrative holistic gynecologist and colleague, recommends a hormone-balancing diet to help the body restore optimum function and fertility, particularly if your infertility is linked to hormone imbalance. This is a low (animal)-fat, high-fiber, nutrient-dense, vegetarian-"style," organic foods regimen that also emphasizes eating plenty of certain foods known for their hormone-balancing properties.

We generally do not recommend dairy products, except for organic, unflavored, unhomogenized yogurt for women with conditions related to estrogen dominance, but we also believe that if you do not suffer from estrogen dominance, organic dairy products in moderation can be fine.

Good Fats You've learned about the bad fats. But there are major types of prostaglandins (E1 and E3), derived from fatty acids that are good. Your body manufactures these prostaglandins from healthy dietary fats that contain omega 3 and 6 essential fatty acids (EFAs). You get these healthy EFAs from ocean fish (sardines, tuna, halibut, mackerel, cod, and salmon), as well as from nonhydrogenated oils made from flax (the best source), safflower, canola, and sesame seeds, wheat germ, walnuts, olives, soybeans, other nuts and seeds, and from organic eggs laid by chickens whose feed is supplemented with the fish oil DHA (docosahexaenoic acid). The omega 3s are found most abundantly in flaxseeds and ocean fish. Good-quality omega 6 fatty acids are easier to get from food: most vegetables, as well as from walnut oil, macadamia oil, sesame oil, hazelnut oil, black currant oil, primrose oil, and borage oil. This is why most people are well supplied with the omega 6 fatty acids but deficient in the omega 3 fatty acids. The E1 series of prostaglandins that your body makes from these food sources may promote blood flow to your pelvic organs. The E3 series of prostaglandins produce an anti-inflammatory effect throughout the body. In order for your body to manufacture these healthy prostaglandins, you also must consume high enough levels of magnesium, B_6, and zinc. Although we recommend ocean fish, according to TCM dietary theory, which considers all foods as either "yin" ("cold") or "yang" ("hot"), raw fish—as in sushi and sashimi—is considered "yin" or "cold" and may not be optimal for fertility. Another choice is to sprinkle two tablespoons of ground flaxseeds on meals each day. Be sure to keep the flaxseed oil and flaxseeds refrigerated, as they turn rancid easily.

Dairy and Meat Products If you eat meat and dairy, choose organic dairy products and meat from free-range animals, because they are allowed to roam freely and are not fed grain contaminated with pesticides and insecticides. Eating small amounts of these lean meats should not cause health problems in most people, and, according to TCM dietary theory, lamb is considered helpful in achieving fertility and boosting virility in men.

Fruit and Veggies The reason why ocean fish may be a source of good fats is because they feed on algae rich in healthy essential fatty acids. A lot of leafy greens are high in these same healthy essential fats, as well as calcium, and you should make them an important part of your diet. According to TCM dietary theory, eating your vegetables lightly cooked is preferable to raw in salads. Uncooked vegetables are thought to be overly "yin" and "cold," thus predisposing you to a "cold" or infertile uterus. Include adequate portions of the following foods in your diet:

- Onions, garlic, the garlic shoot, leeks, chives, and scallions contain potent antioxidants that help prevent free radical damage to body tissue. These pungent "warm" foods are often recommended by TCM practitioners to enhance fertility and counter a "cold uterus," which we discuss more fully later on in this chapter.

- Turnips, parsnips, beets, carrots, and other root vegetables contain antioxidant bioflavonoids and carotenoids (substances that give them various colors). If grown organically, root vegetables additionally contain calcium, magnesium, phosphorus, zinc, iron, and trace minerals—important hormone builders.
- Many vegetables and fruits contain vitamin C, which helps prevent miscarriages, and evidence suggests this water-soluble vitamin also supports adrenal gland and hormone function. Citrus fruit are particularly rich in this important nutrient as well as bioflavonoids that work together for your maximum benefit.

Each bioflavenoid and carotenoid targets a different organ, so one way to make sure that you're getting your essential nutrients from fruit and vegetables is to eat at least six or as many different-colored vegetables and fruit per day as possible.

Nuts and Seeds Seeds (especially flaxseeds) and nuts are a highly nutritious food source packed with high amounts of vitamins and healthy essential fatty acids and high-quality, concentrated, nonanimal protein. Flaxseeds also contain phytoestrogenic substances called lignans that help balance estrogen levels by competing for estrogen-receptor sites against the body's potentially harmful natural estrogens and the even more dangerous xenoestrogens found in chemicals.

Healthy Carbs If fibroids or endometriosis are reducing your fertility, carbs can be a problem if they have what is known as a high-glycemic index. This means that the body identifies and reacts to these carbs as if they were pure sugar, creating excess insulin production that can lead to further hormonal imbalance. If that's your problem, avoid carbs and other foods with a high-glycemic index, even if they're whole grain. These starchy foods include potatoes, yams, sweet potatoes, and flour products such as pasta, breads, cereals, and pastries.

Low-glycemic grains are not only less likely to cause an insulin surge, they also are more alkaline and gluten free. These whole grains also provide a natural form of vitamin E (tocopherol complex), which is essential for smooth reproductive function and works as an effective antioxidant to protect body cells from merging with oxygen or being oxidized, which can destroy them. Vitamin E–rich foods also benefit the pituitary gland. Other foods containing plenty of vitamin E include soybeans, peanuts, asparagus, salmon, spinach, nuts, sunflower seeds, and oils made from sunflower seeds, safflower seeds, almonds, sesame seeds, peanuts, and olives.

Eat plenty of zinc-rich sunflower, pumpkin, and sesame seeds to support hormone production and balance. Gypsies have been eating pumpkin seeds for centuries to balance hormone levels and maintain healthy gynecological function. Myth has it that women in ancient Babylonia nibbled on sesame seed confections to increase fertility. You can do the same by filling a small plastic bag with seeds, so you always have a healthy snack on hand.

It's difficult to get enough vitamin E from food alone, especially if you're older, so the next chapter will give you guidelines on taking vitamin E supplements.

Whole grains also provide lots of B vitamins, which are essential for a healthy nervous system, which, in turn, protects reproductive health. The Bs also boost testosterone levels, a "male" sex hormone also present in females—although in far lower levels—that is responsible for a healthy libido. You must consume adequate amounts of *all* the Bs, because they work together, and low levels of just one B vitamin impairs the ability of the others to do their jobs. All whole grain foods contain high levels of B complex vitamins, so avoid the high-glycemic grains and eat plenty of alkalinizing grains such as brown, long grain, basmati, and wild rice, as well as millet, buckwheat, and oats.

Legumes Beans and peas are good complex carbohydrates that tend to alkalinize rather than acidify the body and also contain the hormone-balancing lignans that act as harmless, mild estrogens to counter more harmful estrogens.

> Warning: A diet heavy in soy can cause low thyroid function, which, as you know can cause infertility. Soy also contains phytates, substances also found in grains and spinach, which can interfere with mineral absorption. A balanced diet, however, will prevent these problems. We can conclude from this that while small amounts of soy are good, larger amounts are not necessarily better. Some women who eat soy with every meal soon start complaining about bloating and stomach cramps.

Pure Water Our bodies are approximately 70 percent water, and all our body fluids depend on sufficient water intake in order to circulate and function properly. We need water to make our blood, urine, lymph, digestive juices, and perspiration. Water also helps cleanse our livers and kidneys, allowing our bodies to excrete hormones efficiently.

In the TCM and other Eastern medical traditions, "dryness" in the pelvis, with an associated reduced level of energy flow, is thought to lead to the condition of "stagnation" that helps create infertility. Many experts suggest that we each drink one ounce of water for every 2 pounds of our body weight each day. That means that a 120-pound woman needs to take in at least sixty ounces of water a day. In other words, don't wait until you are thirsty to drink water. Mineral water is a good choice because, not surprisingly, it is a great source of minerals.

TRADITIONAL CHINESE MEDICINE'S FERTILITY DIET

TCM is an ancient tradition that is mostly anecdotal, and some of the theories have been verified by science only recently. While substantial theory backs TCM recommendations for fertility, you should be warned that it is not scientific and there is almost no research proof we can quote. However, we will share the theory and recommendations with you all the same.

First, as we mentioned earlier, as part of its yin and yang theory, TCM categorizes food items as "yin" ("cold"), "yang" ("hot"), or "neutral," which is the case for the majority of foods. This system of categorization is based on the nature and energy of a particular food; it has nothing to do with the food's temperature or whether it is cooked or raw, although raw foods are more likely to be categorized as "cold." Since TCM generally believes that "blood" is essential to fertility and that blood is "warm," a woman who has difficulty bearing young is diagnosed as having a "cold" uterus. Therefore this woman should avoid "cold" and raw foods and eat more "warming" foods such as mutton and stimulating spices such as pepper and turmeric. Following the same logic, TCM dietary theory recommends eating red meat or drinking beef broth because blood is an essential part of fertility. In our practice, we follow a TCM approach when we recommend avoiding raw and cold foods, including salads and iced drinks, and including more spices in the diet. However, we are oversimplifying the subject in this discussion a bit because the optimal diet must also take into account your body type (whether you tend to be yin or yang), the season (winter is cold, while summer is hot), as well as other factors.

We cannot here go into an extensive discussion of the yin and yang nature of foods, TCM dietary theory, and an exhaustive list of all foods, but these are some examples of "cold-cool" foods to avoid and "hot-warm" foods you can enjoy while enhancing fertility:

- Cold foods: Bamboo shoots, bananas, clams, crab, grapefruit, lettuce, seaweed, water chestnuts, watercress, watermelon
- Cool foods: Apples, bean curd, button mushrooms, cucumber, lettuce, mung beans, pears, spinach, strawberries, tomatoes
- Neutral foods: Apricots, beef, beets, Chinese greens, carrots, celery, corn, eggs, honey, most grains—including bread, rice, potatoes
- Warm foods: Brown sugar, black tea, cherries,

chicken, chives, dates, ham, leeks, mutton, peaches, raspberries, durians, scallions, wine
- Hot foods: Chinese green onions, garlic, ginger, peppers, onions

You should also keep in mind that certain tastes such as sour, salty, and bitter are associated with yin and should be avoided. Pungent foods are usually yang. For those of you who are interested in pursuing this theoretical approach to fertility more formally, we advise you to keep a food diary and consult a knowledgeable TCM practitioner who can review your diet for yin and yang balance while also taking into account your body type.

HOW TO EAT

How you eat is as important as what you eat, because it can affect how efficiently your body uses the nutrients you're taking in. Ensure that your body absorbs the maximum amount of benefit from your food by following these tips on how, where, and when to eat:

- Eat smaller amounts of food more frequently to prevent obesity and stabilize metabolism and blood sugar levels. Try four or five small meals a day instead of three large ones.
- Chew your food thoroughly so you can digest nutrients completely.
- Eat in calm, stress-free settings that allow your digestive tract to perform its job more efficiently.

- Do not eat when you are not hungry because you have not finished digesting the previous meal.
- Do not retain digested foods intentionally. This is an important TCM principle, and it means you should not suppress the urge to belch, pass gas, urinate, or have bowel movements.
- Don't eat on the run. Stress actually impairs your body's ability to absorb and use nutrients.

Try to gradually introduce into your diet the healthy changes you've learned about in this chapter so the process will be easier, even enjoyable. Over time, your taste in food will become more sensitive and refined, and you will be much healthier.

Chapter 9

Boost Your Fertility with Natural Herbs, Vitamins, Supplements, and Over-the-Counter (OTC) Medicines

Not that long ago, diseases associated with nutrient deficiencies, such as scurvy and rickets, were common in the West because most doctors did not understand the connection between diet and disease and dysfunction. Now we know that supplementing our diet with specific vitamins, minerals, herbs, and other substances can protect health and work significant changes in our bodies, including enhancing fertility.

TCM HERBAL THEORY

Herbal remedies have been used in China for perhaps three thousand years and began to be consolidated into a system of medicine about two thousand years ago. The properties of about six thousand herbs are described in the traditional medical literature, and more than five hundred are still used in routine clinical practice. Some are herbs and seasonings—

mint, honeysuckle, cinnamon, ginger, garlic, cilantro, and licorice—we can grow ourselves or buy as groceries. Others—yarrow, rhubarb, gentian, aconite, and yellow vetch—are folk medicines that became well known in the West after Europeans traveled to China in the eighteenth century. Still others—notopterygium, bupleurum, and atractylodes—are more exotic, and some TCM ingredients are even derived from a variety of sources that are decidedly "nonherbal"—animals, marine life, minerals, insects, and worms, to name just a few.

TCM explains the healing properties of herbs with the philosophical theory of correspondences, in which an intricate network of correspondences links all things and all forces together, so that like acts on like and opposing forces balance each other. In this way, an herb designated as "hot" would be used to treat a condition classified as "cold."

Western scientific theory proposes that plants have evolved to produce a great variety of pharmacologically active chemicals as a survival mechanism—attracting insects and animals to graze on them and thereby transport their seeds. The medicinal properties of herbs are confirmed by the fact that many pharmaceutical medicines are derived from plants, for example, white willow bark, the source for aspirin.

NATURE'S HERBAL MEDICINE CHEST

All herbologists agree on one point: expectant women must be especially cautious when taking herbs because they can disrupt a pregnancy. We are very careful in prescribing herbs for infertility and, in most instances, suggest that herbs be taken only for the two weeks after your menses, since you can be pregnant without being aware of it. Since some herbs that boost fertility can also cause a miscarriage, many practitioners do not use herbs at all when treating infertile patients. If you are not sure an herb is safe, don't take it. In fact, only three herbs are generally considered safe for pregnant women by all experts in the field: garlic (*Allium sativum*) in small amounts, cooked in food; ginger (*Zingiber officinalis*) for morning sickness, and spearmint (*Mentha spicata*) for morning sickness.

That said, many medicinal herbs exhibit beneficial effects on both the male and female reproductive systems. If you are certain you are not pregnant or if you have fibroids, endometriosis, or any other hormone-imbalance condition that needs to be treated before you try again to become pregnant, the right herbs can be helpful because they can increase or decrease production levels of reproductive hormones and balance the entire endocrine system.

Today, we are rediscovering time-tested natural herbal teas and fluid extracts, and even putting botanical supplements in tablets and capsules. Still, a very small percentage of the plant species on the earth has been studied for medicinal properties, since studies to verify the healing powers of herbs would cost many millions of dollars. What drug company would underwrite costs to verify the strengthening and healing properties of a substance that grows wild, as a gift from nature—a substance it cannot patent and profit from?

This is why many of the claims made for herbal healing have been based on anecdotal clinical evidence rather than on scientifically sanctioned clinical trials. Although more studies of herbs are being conducted today than ever before, we often have to rely on the reports of herbal practitioners past and present.

Because the herbal healing system employed by practitioners of traditional Chinese medicine is so complex, you should generally not treat yourself with Chinese herbs. It is also crucial that your TCM practitioner be well versed in how Chinese herbs should be used to enhance fertility. Again, this is because some of the herbs used to prepare your body for pregnancy can also cause a miscarriage if you are already pregnant.

Herbs can be divided into several basic groups: nutritive, carminative, astringent, disinfectant, and tonic. For our purpose, which is rebalancing hormones and strengthening the reproductive glands in preparation for pregnancy, the herbs we use to support and stimulate hormone and organ function are certain of the tonic herbs.

> If you are potentially fertile, it may be safer to take herbs only for the two weeks after your menses (days one to fourteen). You may resume taking herbs once your pregnancy test is negative after day fourteen. Once you are pregnant or may be pregnant, stop taking all herbs and herbal remedies unless at the advice of a medical expert. Never mix herbs and fertility drugs unless under the specific guidance and direction of an herbal specialist and your fertility doctor.

Notable Female Tonic Herbs

Tonic herbs—the safest of all herbs—are generally nontoxic and usually can be used over the long term. They can be taken either individually or in compound remedies in which several herbs work together synergistically to strengthen and tone your body. Tonics are available as capsules, tinctures, decoctions, or as an infusion or tea. The following tonic herbs, commonly thought to enhance female fertility, are sometimes used by TCM and other holistic and alternative medical practitioners to boost or balance hormone production in women:

Black Cohosh (*Cimicifuga racemosa*) Also known as squawroot, black cohosh (the roots) has been used by Native Americans for centuries. Because of its estrogenlike effects it has been historically given during childbirth as a preparation for delivery. More recently, it is frequently being used as a natural hormone replacement for menopausal women. Since, it can reduce LH levels, it may act as a regulator and suppress ovulation. It is also thought to strengthen the uterus.

Dose: For a tea, boil 2 tsp. of dried roots in a pint of water. Take 2 or 3 tsp. six times a day. Take 5 to 30 drops of the fluid extract in a cup of water once a day, or take 2 to 3 capsules a day.

Safety issues: If there is the slightest chance that you may be pregnant, do not use this herb because it can cause a miscarriage. Also, very large doses can cause symptoms of poisoning.

Chaste Tree Berry (*Vitex agnus-castus*) This herb has been used in Europe for two thousand years and is perhaps the most well researched Western herb relating to female hormone regulation. It is thought to regulate menstrual irregularities, soothe premenstrual tension, enhance female fertility, as well as being useful for PCOS. It usually takes three to four months to see some effect from using it. Chaste tree berry may be particularly helpful in cases of infertility where a woman has no periods, irregular periods, long cycles, and, of course, luteal phase defect (a deficiency of progesterone during the luteal phase of the menstrual cycle).

Research shows that for menstrual irregularities due to

luteal phase defect, chaste tree berry is thought to work on the hypothalamus and pituitary glands by increasing LH levels and inhibiting the release of FSH, which in turn leads to enhanced progesterone levels. Chaste tree berry also inhibits prolactin release, and high prolactin levels sometimes cause infertility.

Dose: In general, 60 drops of standardized tincture or 400–500 mg of the standardized extract containing 0.5 percent agnusides may be used once daily, although individual dosage requirements may vary. It can be used for up to eighteen months or until you become pregnant, but actual dosing depends on the particular patient, so your best bet is to work with an herbalist.

Safety issues: Though there are generally none, absolutely avoid this herb during IVF as it may cause ovarian hyperstimulation. If you are taking oral contraceptives, use chaste tree berry only under a doctor's supervision.

Red Clover (*Trifolium pratense*) This is a Western perennial whose flower is traditionally used for cough and skin problems. Some noted herbalists, such as Susun Weed, consider this to be the single most important herb to establish fertility. It contains several weak estrogenlike compounds (phytoestrogens), as well as volatile oils and other ingredients. Red clover is frequently included in over-the-counter supplements marketed to enhance female fertility.

Dose: The fresh or dried flower is used. The usual recommended dose is 4 g taken as a capsule or 1/2 tsp. of a 1:1 liquid extract taken three times a day.

Safety issues: red clover is generally considered safe when used as prescribed.

Dong Quai (*Angelica sinensis*) An excellent tonic for female reproductive glands and organs, this is one of the most well known of Chinese herbs for women's health. Dong quai has been used by traditional Asian healers for many centuries to cure many female disorders, and most commonly for relieving menopausal symptoms and painful menstrual cramping.

Dong quai is widely available in health food stores, Chinese herbal pharmacies, and through mail order in capsule and tincture forms. It is frequently found in compound tonics prescribed by both Chinese and Western herbalists. Some compound formulas combine dong quai with chaste tree berry, which may help balance hormone levels, thereby ensuring healthy function of the reproductive organs and glands.

Dose: You can take 20 drops of dong quai twice a day. In its other forms, follow the dose instructions on the bottle label.

Safety issues: Though it is generally considered safe, some of the chemical components in dong quai can interact with sunlight and cause a rash.

Evening Primrose (*Oenothera biennis*) The oil derived from this North American herb has been traditionally known to relieve breast pain and menstrual pains. It is a rich source of both linoleic acid and gamma-linoleic acid (GLA). GLA can be converted in the body to a hormonelike substance called prostaglandin E1, which has anti-inflammatory properties and may act as a blood vessel dilator. Evening primrose oil is also thought to improve the quality of the cervical mucus, which aids the sperm in swimming through to the uterus and the egg. If your cervical mucus is thick or brown or if you are very dry or lack cervical mucus, you may consider using this herb.

Dose: Evening primrose should be taken from time of menses through mid-cycle. You can take up to 3,000 mg of the oil a day.

Safety issues: As with most herbs, you must be extra careful if you become pregnant. Use of evening primrose oil during pregnancy can increase the risk for complications.

Licorice (*Glycyrrhiza glabra*) This herb, native to the Mediterranean area and Asia, appears to modulate hormonal production and metabolism. Known as "the great harmonizer" in Chinese medicine, its tasty root sweetens many tonic formulas, and is also a good anti-inflammatory, tonifier, and energizer, particularly for weak kidneys and adrenal glands, mainly by virtue of its steroidlike active ingredients, which are mainly saponins, as well as a vast array of over forty different other ingredients. Licorice also contains estrogenlike compounds (phytoestrogens) and has a mild estrogenic effect making it useful in easing PMS and menopausal symptoms. Reports from Japan show positive results in the use of licorice in treating menstrual problems related to elevated androgen levels such as seen in PCOS patients.

Dose: Licorice root is available in whole form in health food stores and Asian herbal stores. It is also widely available in tea, capsule, and tincture form. The dose is based on the content level of its active ingredients, particularly glycyrrhizin.

Safety issues: Licorice is potent but not an entirely benign herb. Do not take it if you have hypertension or a history of kidney dysfunction, or if you are taking a digitalis preparation. If more than 3 g are taken per day, for more than six weeks, licorice can cause water and sodium retention, hypertension, and other problems.

Red Raspberry (*Rubus ideaus*) Red raspberry leaves strengthen and tone the uterus, and help relieve female problems of almost all kinds through a wonderfully soothing action. Although some herbalists believe red raspberry is one of the few herbs that can be used throughout pregnancy, the usual precaution should apply. Among red raspberry's many benefits to women are reducing overly heavy menstrual flow, easing uterine cramps and labor pains, and toning the uterus in preparation for gestating a child. Tea made from it is said to help prevent miscarriage and morning sickness, but you should use it only under a doctor's advice (especially during the last two months of pregnancy) because, in some instances, red raspberry has been associated with premature labor. Red raspberry also has astringent and cleansing properties, making it an excellent herb for post-childbirth recovery.

Dose: Red raspberry is available in bulk, tea bags, and, for healing purposes, in capsule and tincture forms. The usual dose for the tea is 3 cups a day. In tincture form, take 1 tsp. up to three times a day. Otherwise, follow the dose instructions on the bottle label.

Sarsaparilla (*Smilax officinalis*) Anecdotal reports indicate that sarsaparilla root and berries tone the reproductive organs and glands and may be useful for amenorrhea. Traditional American herbalists recommend taking sarsaparilla tonics for a few weeks in spring and fall as a regular practice.

Dose: You can take this herb in tea form, capsule, or extract as general daily tonic, for months at a time.

Safety issues: There are generally none if it is used sparingly. Excessive doses can lead to intestinal irritation or kidney impairment.

White Willow (*Salix alba*) This may be the least appreciated fertility-enhancing herb, yet, ironically, it is the best documented. Let me explain why: White willow is also known as "herbal aspirin," because it contains salicin, an element your body converts into salicylic acid (aspirin), which quite possibly has all the benefits aspirin gives to fertility. (See pages 201–203 for a more thorough discussion on baby aspirin.) In addition, white willow can be used to enhance the uterine lining, improve IVF success, and reduce recurrent miscarriages.

Dose: The herb is available in many forms and should be standardized to salicin content. The equivalent of 40 mg of salicin daily should be used for fertility.

Safety issues: Although it is thought to be gentler than aspirin on the stomach, white willow can thin the blood and irritate the stomach. Those who are allergic to aspirin should avoid taking it. Those who have a bleeding disorder or history of peptic ulcer should consult a medical professional before taking this herb on their own.

Many other herbs are mentioned in folklore as potentially helpful in promoting female fertility, although the claims have not been confirmed as yet by scientific studies. Some examples include false unicorn root, stinging nettles (*Urtica dioica*), damiana (*Turnera diffusa*), partridgeberry (*Mitchella repens*), liferoot (*Senecio aureus*), and fenugreek (*Trigonella foenum-graecum*). You should also know that specific herbs are thought to have antifertility effects in women and are therefore used to regulate fertility. These include wild carrot or Queen Anne's lace (*Daucus carota*), wild yam (*Dioscorea villosa*), and pennyroyal (*Mentha pulegium*), to name a few. This is why you shouldn't take herbs while attempting to get pregnant unless you are working with an expert and every medical practitioner on your "fertility team" is aware of what you are taking. The same goes for your partner: many herbs are advertised for enhancing male sexual performance and quite a few also improve sperm function. However, even a common herb such as Saint-John's-wort, which is commonly used to treat depression, has been shown to depress sperm production and motility. Your best bet is to consult a professional herbologist before using any herbs on your own.

Even ginseng (*Panax ginseng*), an Eastern herb surrounded by myths of its power as a tonic as well as scientific research supporting its effectiveness in boosting sperm production and motility, recently was shown to be potentially detrimental to fertility. Researchers from Hong Kong have found evidence that ginsenoside Rb1—one of the principal active components of ginseng—can cause abnormalities in embryos. Dr. Louis Chan and colleagues at the Chinese University of Hong Kong, Prince of Wales Hospital, tested ginsenoside Rb1 in various concentrations on nine-day-old rat embryos. They found that embryos exposed to more than 30 mcg per 1 ml of ginsenoside Rb1 had significantly low developmental scores. The embryos specifically had lower scores for heart, limbs, and eye development and flexion. At the highest dose of 50 mcg, the embryos were also significantly shorter in body length and had fewer somites (muscle precursor cells).

TCM COMPOUND HERBAL REMEDIES

TCM herbs are generally prescribed in a compound remedy so the herbs can create a synergistic effect that balances and stimulates particular elements of the mind-body system. Tonics promote strength, energy, reproductive function, and a hardy, balanced nervous system. The right compound tonic can be wonderful preventative treatment to enhance vitality and well-being, and it can also be part of a program to build up your fertility. While several traditional herbal tonic formulas are available over the counter, in health food stores, and in Chinese herbal shops, again, do not take them unless they are prescribed by a knowledgeable TCM practitioner.

Examples of Herbal Remedies Commonly Prescribed for Each Infertility-Linked Type of Imbalance

Although the herbal remedies prescribed by TCM practitioners are many and diverse—far too numerous to list in this book—the compound formulas that follow are commonly prescribed according to the particular type of fertility-linked imbalance.

For kidney yin and yang deficiency:

- Two Immortals formula (Damiana and Gotu Kola formula). Ingredients include damiana (Turnera diffusa), gotu kola (Radix hydrocotyle asiatica), schizandra (wu wei zi), oystershell (mu li), morinda (ba ji tian), epimedium (yin yang huo), tang kuei (dang gui), ligustrum (nu zhen zi), eclipta (han lian cao), red dates (da zao), pseudostellaria (tai zi shen), anemarrhena (zhi mu), phellodendron (zhi gan cao), baked licorice (zhi gan cao), eight moon fruit (ba yue zha), and scrophalia (xuan shen).

- Conceptive Pill, with modifications. Ingredients include 15 g salvia (dan shen); 12 g each human placenta (zi he che) and prepared rehmannia (shu di huang); 9 g each atractylodes (big head) (bai zhu), poria (fu ling), white peony (bai shao yao), ligusticum (chuan xiong), tang kuei (dang gui), dodder seed (tusi zi), eucommia bark (du zhong), cyperus root (ziang fu zi), and prepared licorice (gan cao); and 1.5 g prickly ash bark (hua jiao).

For blood deficiency:

- Bupleurum Liver Coursing Powder (also called Bupleurum Powder to Spread the Liver; Chai Hu Shu Gan San). This quickens the blood flow, resolves depression, and relieves pain. It consists of 6 g each bupleurum (chai hu) and tangerine peel (chen pi); 4.5 g each ligusticum (chuan xiong), cyperus (ziang fu zi), bitter orange (zhi ke), and peony (bai shao); and 1.5 g honey-fried licorice.
- Conceptive Decoction by Soothing the Liver. This also dispels stagnant blood. It includes 15 g white peony (bai shao yao) and 9 g each tang kuei (dang gui), atractylodes (big head) (bai zhu), poria (fu ling), and snake gourd root (tian hua fen).

You should not use these or any other herbal formulas unless you first have been carefully diagnosed and then given a personalized formula prepared by an experienced TCM herbalist. In our practice, if a patient is susceptible to weakness or dysfunction in the reproductive organs and glands or is over forty, we sometimes prescribe a tonic formula to prepare the body for conception and gestation before she attempts to become pregnant. Again, once you are pregnant, or suspect that you may be pregnant, stop taking all herbs immediately.

FERTILITY-ENHANCING VITAMINS AND SUPPLEMENTS

Traditional Chinese medicine does not employ vitamin or mineral supplements, as do Western alternative and complementary health practitioners. Vitamins and supplements are vital, however, and, in many aspects, much better studied than herbs. We certainly recommend that our patients supplement with vitamins and minerals in their quest to enhance their fertility.

The subject of supplements can be confusing. Supplement manufacturers make wild and extravagant claims, so how can you really know what to take, when to take it, and in what amounts? This chapter gives you guidelines to make the right choices.

> Many of the supplements you'll learn about can be used safely on your own to strengthen and balance your endocrine system and reproductive organs *in preparation* for pregnancy. *If you are actively trying to become pregnant, you must make your doctor aware of everything you are taking, because some substances may have interactions with fertility drugs or should not be continued after you become pregnant.*

Why Take Supplements?

Some people do not see the value in taking supplements, especially if they believe their diet provides them with everything they need. But there are many reasons why supplements may be a good idea for you, especially if you're trying to get pregnant.

Your diet is probably worse than you think. According to some studies, less than half of all Americans eat the recommended three to five servings of vegetables a day. Even if you think that you eat healthily, your intake of food is likely to fall short in some vitamin or mineral because requirements to prepare your body for optimal fertility may be different. Some of your other food choices—such as fried foods containing harmful fats—may even sabotage your efforts toward a healthy diet. If you eat these, taking antioxidant supplements can help. The point is, virtually every national nutritional study since the sixties has found that people aren't meeting even the *minimum* recommended dietary allowances (RDAs) for nutrients. The bottom line is that the best way to ensure you get the nutrients you need to promote fertility and create a healthy environment for a developing child is to use a smart combination of the right diet and the right supplements.

A small but important study published by a group of Stanford University researchers in the April 2004 issue of the *Journal of Reproductive Medicine*, shows that just taking vitamins and supplements, without other interventions, dramatically promoted fertility. In a double-blind test (where neither subjects nor researchers knew who was taking vitamins and who was taking placebos), thirty women ages twenty-four to forty-six who had tried unsuccessfully to conceive were given either placebos or a vitamin and supplement blend. After five months, five of the fifteen women in the supplement group were pregnant (33 percent), while none of the fifteen women in the placebo group had become pregnant.

Choosing the Right Multivitamin-Mineral Supplement

Nearly all women seeking to become pregnant can benefit from a high-potency multivitamin-mineral supplement that may give fertility a boost. Unfortunately, most gynecologists and fertility specialists are still recommending that women take prenatal vitamins, which are primarily intended to fortify the fetus. Prenatal supplements prepare for pregnancy, but they do not help get you pregnant. What you really need before you are even pregnant is a preconception vitamin. Once you become pregnant, then you can switch to a prenatal vitamin supplement.

If your doctor has recommended that you take a prenatal vitamin supplement and you are trying to conceive, ask the doctor whether you may switch to a preconception vitamin supplement instead. The primary purpose of prenatals is to nourish the fetus in a woman who is already pregnant.

Table 9.1 Recommended Daily Amounts for a Preconception Multivitamin-Mineral

Vitamin/Mineral	Amount
Vitamin D	200–300 IU
Vitamin E	10–50 IU
Vitamin C	100–250 mg
Calcium	250–300 mg
Copper	2–3 mg
Zinc	15–25 mg
Folic acid	800 mcg or more
Iron	2 mg or more
Magnesium	250–500 mg
Manganese	1–2 mg
Selenium	50–100 mcg
B vitamins, including B_1, B_2, B_3, B_6, B_{12}*	varying amounts

*Most of the Bs are readily available in a balanced diet. These vitamins are not proven to bolster fertility, but may be included in a supplement for general health and fertility.

The recommendations in Table 9.1 are based on extensive research we've conducted, on veterinary and human data, to investigate the optimally balanced vitamin and mineral supplement intake for increasing fertility. In fact, the amino acid L-arginine is all-important, as we will explain, and should be present in a preconception supplement in an amount of no less than 2 g per day.

Quality of vitamins and supplements varies from manufacturer to manufacturer, so keep in mind the following guidelines when choosing a multivitamin or mineral or any vitamin or mineral supplement:

- Don't buy supplements labeled "time-release." These contain clays that slow the absorption in your digestive tract. Even if you notice no adverse reactions at first, repeated exposure over time can cause you to become sensitive to the clays.
- Avoid one-a-day brands. These brands deliver excessively high levels of the supplement in a single pill or capsule. It's better to space out your supplement intake over the day, taking one with each meal.
- If you are undergoing fertility drug treatment at the same time, make sure you do not use a supplement that also contains herbs with hormonal actions.
- Look on the bottle label of your mineral supplements for the amino acids aspartate, picolinate, malate, or citrate. Since experts estimate that as little as 10 percent of most mineral supplements are actually absorbed, a good supplement attaches its mineral components to the above amino acids to increase absorbability.
- Never take a heavy-duty vitamin-mineral supplement on an empty stomach; this can cause cramps and nausea, and inhibit your body's ability to absorb the nutrients. Food enhances the absorption of supplements. This is especially important with fat-soluble antioxidants and nutrients (such as vitamins D and E), which require a little fat or oil for absorption. You don't need to eat a lot of fat; just a spoonful of peanut butter or olive oil is enough. Always take a supplement either mid-meal or within twenty minutes of finishing a meal.
- Take capsules instead of tablets whenever possible. Capsules release their contents faster than tablets.

- Don't keep an open bottle of supplements more than six to nine months, and keep supplement bottles in the refrigerator, especially if they contain fats or oils.

Special Fertility Boosters

In our practice, depending on a patient's particular condition, we may recommend certain vitamins, minerals, and other supplements that are particularly helpful in correcting infertility.

L-arginine This all-important amino acid occurs naturally in your body and has been scientifically studied to promote fertility in both males and females. It works by being converted into nitric oxide (NO) as it is being metabolized by the body. Nitric oxide improves blood flow to the pelvis, nourishing the ovaries (and eggs) and the endometrial lining. Stanford University researchers demonstrated a 40 percent increased pregnancy rate in otherwise infertile women who were given a vitamin supplement containing L-arginine. In addition, L-arginine is potentially helpful during IVF.

In an Italian study published in the July 1999 issue of *Human Reproduction*, seventeen patients who were characterized as "poor responders" and had failed previous IVF cycles were given L-arginine in addition to standard IVF. Another group of seventeen "poor responders" received standard IVF only. The L-arginine treated group experienced a lower cancellation rate, an increased number of eggs collected, and an increased number of embryos transferred. Significant blood flow improvement in the pelvis was also observed by ultrasound for the women in the L-arginine-supplemented group.

Three pregnancies were registered in the L-arginine patients; no pregnancies were observed in the standard treatment group.

The same Italian study found that L-arginine may be equally useful for subfertile men to enhance sperm function. The therapeutic dose for men ranges from 2 g a day, at minimum, to as much as 16 g a day.

Gamma-linolenic Acid (GLA) GLAs are essential fatty acids that protect reproductive health and prevent many ailments, including those that impair fertility. You can take one to two tablespoons per day of cold-pressed flaxseed oil either alone or drizzled on your vegetables. Or you can take a mixed essential fatty acid complex capsule that gives you a balance of omega 3s, 6s, and 9s—one capsule in morning and in evening. All brands contain from 500 to 1,000 mg per capsule.

OVER-THE-COUNTER MEDICINES THAT BOOST FERTILITY

Because we practice TCM and alternative medicine, many people assume we must be against drugs. Actually, we are not against anything—advanced technologies or medicines—as long as they help you achieve your goal and do not harm your well-being. In fact, some simple, over-the-counter medicines are quite helpful for infertility.

Baby Aspirin This medicine is salicylic acid, one of the oldest of the chemical drugs known to modern man, because it derived originally from the white willow tree. While aspirin may seem to be a lowly and ubiquitous remedy, many people underestimate its many therapeutic properties, which range from healing sunburn to preventing heart attacks and strokes.

Aspirin is not just for fevers and aches or pains, and its unique ability to improve blood flow and function as an anti-inflammatory gives it a facility for improving many conditions that hamper infertility. For example, one of the less common causes of miscarriage is the so-called recurrent miscarriage syndrome (RMS). The most common singular problem in women with RMS is a blood-clotting defect that can sometimes be treated successfully with baby aspirin and other anti-coagulant medications. Baby aspirin has another fertility use: it can improve the uterine lining, which can lead to a successful pregnancy. In 2000, researchers from Taiwan reported in the medical literature on 236 women who suffered from infertility and had thin uterine linings. These women were divided into two groups, a group that took aspirin and a group that did not. In the group that experienced aspirin therapy, there were significantly higher percentages of thicker and better endometrium (46.5 percent vs. 26.2 percent) and pregnancy rates (18.4 percent vs. 9.0 percent). Another study from Israel in the same year reported on baby aspirin's benefits in 52 consecutive women who had suffered repeated IVF failures and had evidence of autoimmunity in their blood, such as exhibiting anti-cardiolipin antibodies (ACA), antinuclear antibodies (ANA), anti-double-stranded (ds) DNA, rheumatoid factor (RF), and/or lupus anticoagulant (LAC). These patients were treated with a protocol that included 100 mg of aspirin starting four weeks before induction of ovulation, and they achieved an astounding 32.7 percent pregnancy rate. We recommend a dose of 80 mg (the standard amount in one baby aspirin) once a day.

A research group in Argentina conducted a double-blind, randomized controlled trial to assess the role of baby aspirin in assisted reproduction. One hundred and forty-nine patients undergoing IVF were randomly assigned to take low-dose (100 mg) aspirin or a placebo. At the conclusion of the study, the researchers found more eggs retrieved (16.2 vs. 8.6) and better serum hormonal levels and pelvic blood flow in the aspirin-treated patients. Most important, the pregnancy rate (45 percent vs. 28 percent) and implantation rate (17.8 percent vs. 9.2 percent) were significantly much better in the aspirin-treated women. The researchers concluded that low-dose aspirin significantly improves ovarian responsiveness, uterine and ovarian blood flow velocity, implantation, and pregnancy rates in IVF patients. These results were published in the May 1999 issue of *Fertility and Sterility*.

One word of caution before you rush out and start taking aspirin. Aspirin is a drug and not devoid of potential side effects. Even baby aspirin can thin the blood and cause bruising, as well as serious hemorrhage. Do not take aspirin if you have a bleeding disorder or a history of peptic ulcer, unless advised by your physician. You should always inform and seek the approval of your fertility physician before taking any supplements and drugs.

Guaifenesin A common ingredient found in over-the-counter cough syrups, guaifenesin is thought to promote cervical mucus. Reports on this benefit appeared in the medical literature as early as twenty years ago, and there is even a published report on the case of a forty-six-year-old woman with high FSH who underwent a successful pregnancy after using guaifenesin. There are certainly no known side effects from its use. The usual dose would be one to two teaspoons of a guaifenesin-containing cough medicine, four times a day.

> Warning! Women seeking to conceive should never take more than 5,000 IU daily of vitamin A. In fact, it's best to avoid it altogether, because if you become pregnant, vitamin A can be toxic to the developing embryo. Women with liver problems may be at particular risk for vitamin A toxicity.

Chapter 10

Less Is More: Exercise May Undermine Fertility

Most of us think that exercise is healthy for everyone. Cardiovascular specialists recently issued a recommendation for upping the daily quota of exercise from thirty to sixty minutes of aerobic activity every day in order to protect heart and vascular health. Very few people, and even fewer doctors, would challenge the "fact" that exercise is good for you.

We certainly do not argue that aerobic exercise is unhealthy. Clearly, in many instances it is beneficial, especially for preventing heart disease or obesity. In the past ten years or so, we've seen gyms mushrooming all over this country, especially in cities. It's even trendy nowadays to hit the gym for working out and socializing. However, when it comes to enhancing your fertility, the rule for aerobic exercise is less is actually more. While aerobic exercise can lower fertility, other forms of exercise like yoga or tai chi—what we call fertility-enhancing activities—can actually increase fertility.

WHY LESS EXERCISE IS MORE

The perception that exercise is healthy and beneficial for every single health condition is simply not true. The human species was not built to exercise in spurts the way we do now—for an hour or so at the gym every day or even three times a week. Sure, we were designed to be active, but not necessarily in the form of explosive bursts of activity that are typical of a gym or health club workout. For example, orthopedic physicians know that runners, in particular, commonly suffer injuries to the bones, ligaments, and muscles of their hips, thighs, knees, legs, ankles, and feet from this type of exercise.

Many scientific studies have found a negative correlation between women's ovarian function and exercise. Our clinic patients are usually shocked to learn the following study results: even a young college coed who runs just eight miles a week—the equivalent of only a little over a mile a day or only twenty minutes a day on a treadmill—can experience a lower ovulation rate. Six to 8 percent of women who run eight to ten miles per week will not have a menstrual period for 75 percent (three-quarters) of the year. As you now know, lack of a menstrual period is a reliable sign that no ovulation is taking place. Ovulation is compromised even more severely for runners who log sixty miles per week; approximately 60 percent of these women will have no period at all.

It's clear that the more you exercise, the less fertile you may become. Marathon runners and ballet dancers who don't ovulate are only extreme examples that highlight the issue of exercise and infertility.

You can have regular periods but still suffer from impaired fertility because regular aerobic exercise is setting off body signals that shut down the ovaries. In other words, so-called healthy exercise can send the wrong fertility message to your brain.

As you know from reading about the hormonal chain of command, the brain is ultimately responsible for signaling the ovaries to release an egg each month. When you consider that the act of running and other forms of strenuous exercise were built into our species as a means to avoid danger or to forage for food, then you can appreciate how excessive running or exercising could impede fertility: it cues your deeper consciousness that you live in a place of danger or there's not enough food out there, and, therefore, this is not a good time to reproduce.

As I tell my patients, the brain is literal and doesn't recognize that you are exercising only for health or fun. So, if you are running, your brain can interpret that to mean the environment as hostile to pregnancy. Your brain may then issue signals that move through the hormonal chain of command, telling all hormone players not to release an egg because you're constantly chased by a dangerous beast or trying to escape other dangers. The result is no ovulation, no period—no baby.

Exercise causes fertility problems in other ways, but before we describe each of them, let's take a look at what actually goes on during exercise. Exercise is a combustion phenomenon. This means that during exercise you huff and puff, breathe in lots of oxygen, and burn fuel. That's why exercise helps you lose weight: you burn extra calories and carbohydrates in order to meet the heightened demands on your body. In other words, you burn fuel in the presence of oxygen in order to generate the level of energy exercise requires. It's the same process for a human being, a car engine, an airplane, or anything else that needs to generate energy. Burning oxygen together with fuel generates energy. That's why you feel hot when you exercise. The burning process that generates energy also creates a by-product—waste, whether it's a car putting out exhaust fumes or a human being putting out free radicals and acid. The bodily exhaust that is generated from exercise is what causes your muscles to ache, makes you feel tired, depresses your immune system, and compromises ovarian function.

Now, let's go over the ways exercise affects your fertility:

- Exercise potentially leads to a suppression of ovulation via the hormonal chain of command that starts in the brain.
- Exercise generates a lot of oxygen-free radicals that could potentially damage gametes—the term used for both egg and sperm—in ways similar to the damage it wreaks on other body cells.
- Exercise directs blood flow away from the pelvis and its organs because that blood is being redirected to the muscles that need it. Remember how your mother warned you not to swim or perform other exercise after you ate? She was right. She knew your digestion would suffer because exercise directs blood flow away from your digestive tract, where it's needed to absorb and assimilate food. In the same way, good blood circulation is important to maintaining fertility, so exercise impedes fertility by diverting blood flow away from the pelvis. Blood is particularly necessary because it brings nourishment to cells and carries away waste products.

FERTILITY-ENHANCING ACTIVITIES—NOT EXERCISES

The advice we give women in our practice is that humans are designed biologically to be active, and the right *activities* are helpful. They reduce stress, improve sleep habits, and help the body secrete surplus hormones, thus helping restore the hormone balance necessary for optimum fertility.

The loss of vitality and health that can cause infertility usually takes time. Unfortunately, doctors and other health care givers are seeing more loss of qi, vital life-force energy, in younger people, along with infertility. Since traditional Chinese medicine works to promote balanced movement and flow throughout the mind-body complex, it also includes certain activities or disciplines in concert with acupuncture, diet, herbs, relaxation, and meditation. This holistic treatment package effectively helps overcome chronic fatigue, impotence, low libido, pelvic organ dysfunction, and infertility, along with associated depression and other negative emotional states.

You're probably wondering by now which kinds of activities are okay if I'm trying to conceive.

We always tell our patients that the notion of the right type of physical motion as an essential for life is at the heart of all ancient Asian healing traditions, as seen in the practices of tai chi, qigong (pronounced "chi kung"), yoga, (developed in India), and other disciplines. These are the right *activities* because they are "less aerobic" (generally conducted at a lower heart rate and respiratory rate); because, in essence, they are moving meditations performed with deep, rhythmic breathing that enhance energy flow, level, and balance to improve health and vitality; increase motor skills; eliminate stress; and boost fertility. It is difficult to learn these ancient energy practices on your own, but some people do well with instructional DVDs or videotapes. Your best bet is to find classes for these disciplines in your area. Be sure not to practice these disciplines in their vigorous forms, such as the aerobic or "burning" styles of "power" or ashtanga yoga. We in the West may have come a long way, but we are only just beginning to understand the connection between exercise, health, and fertility.

Naomi was thirty-two years old and beaming with health, but she couldn't get pregnant. When she came in for her initial appointment in 2003, I immediately noticed her athletic qualities: she was tan, toned, and dressed in a tennis outfit and sneakers, with a water bottle in hand and gym bag slung across her shoulder. She told me that she had just come from the gym and apologized for her profuse sweating. She went on to lament that she and her husband couldn't seem to get pregnant although fertility specialists had found nothing wrong. As we talked, I learned that she was from an athletic family. Naomi's father was once a squash champion and she was raised on a philosophy of fitness and sports. Noami was a marathon runner who competed every year in New York City's marathon, in addition to playing tennis regularly and working out almost every day for an hour or more. When I told Naomi that exercise may be damaging her fertility, she literally fell back in the chair. "That's impossible!" she burst out. "No doctor ever told me that! I thought exercise is healthy for you!" I told Naomi that exercise is healthy for certain organs, such as the heart and the lungs, but it was not healthy for her eggs. I reminded her of her past running injuries, and told Naomi to try imagining any of our cousins in the animal kingdom (like a chimp, monkey, or any other primate) running on a treadmill for ninety minutes a day. What in nature could prompt a primate to huff and puff and run nonstop for an hour every day? Only danger, perhaps being chased by another beast. I asked Naomi if she thought the body would consider it wise to become pregnant if one is being chased by beasts every day. She couldn't answer the question, but she said she felt so good after exercising (from the endorphin release that no doubt had literally made Naomi "addicted" to her gym routine) that she was afraid she'd become depressed if she couldn't exercise. I assured Naomi that we did not intend for her to become inactive. Instead, we advised substituting Pilates, yoga, swimming or another less aerobic and less intense form of exercise, as well as learning relaxation techniques while she was trying to get pregnant. We also designed an individual course of acupuncture treatment for Naomi. She followed our advice and, exactly eleven weeks after dropping her gym routine, she was happily pregnant.

Traditional Eastern healers and philosophers have understood the profound relationship between physical activity and fertility for many centuries. That is why certain yoga exercises from ancient India and virtually all the Taoist exercises from ancient China are designed to increase and balance energy flow, in much the same way that acupuncture enhances reproductive health and increases fertility.

After practicing yoga, Taoist postures, or similar activities for a few months, you naturally tune into your body. You become more sensitive to its various workings—the stretch of your muscles, the blood pumping through your vessels—and you begin to take more physical enjoyment in this intricate miracle machine of yours. Your practice is no longer a duty; it becomes your pleasure.

THE FERTILITY BENEFITS OF ENERGY-BALANCING ACTIVITIES

The right activities can affect your fertility as profoundly as acupuncture treatments. You will experience the following benefits:

- More efficient body systems—nervous, immune, digestive, cardiac, and reproductive
- Increased flow of blood, qi, and other substances in the pelvic area
- Better hormone production, including higher testosterone to increase libido in you and your partner, and increased estrogen to promote your fertility
- More endorphins, the body's "feel good" hormones (These natural painkillers promote a feeling of well-being that reduces anxiety and stress and banishes mild depression.)
- More regular menstrual periods and fewer PMS symptoms
- A draining in the prostate of backed-up seminal fluid for your partner
- Increased overall energy

Kegel Pelvic Exercises: A Western Adaptation of Eastern Practices

The pubococcygeus (PC) muscle located in the perineum, between the vagina and anal opening, is directly involved in sexual and reproductive function, so all traditional Asian disciplines offer movements designed to tone and sensitize this muscle to increase circulation, libido, reproductive health, and fertility in the general pelvic area.

We in the West have boiled down the myriad of exercises Asian disciplines offer for strengthening pelvic organs and muscles into a single exercise, although it is quite effective when practiced regularly—Kegels. "Kegeling" involves rhythmically contracting and relaxing the PC muscle, as if you were trying to stop the flow of urine. Although they usually are prescribed to women, Kegel exercises also benefit men.

One great thing about Kegeling is these exercises can be done anywhere, at any time, in front of anyone, and no one will be the wiser. Establishing a regular Kegeling routine is up to you. You even can "trick" yourself into a daily routine by linking Kegel sessions to other daily activities. Here are some suggestions:

- While showering or in the bath (If women combine Kegeling with a fifteen-minute soak in a saltwater bath—using one cup sea salt to a full tub of warm water—they are also cultivating a healthy bacterial environment in the vagina.)
- While brushing and flossing (The advantage of linking these two chores is that most of us do not clean our teeth long enough. This helps you to do both beneficial activities longer. It's also a good exercise in coordination—like patting your head and rubbing your tummy at the same time.)
- Before or after every meal
- While waiting for a traffic light to change, or to pay a bridge or tunnel toll

- While watching television
- While on hold during a phone call
- While standing in line at the bank, movies, or supermarket

How Often to Kegel Ideally, Kegeling could be done three times a day, but do not assign yourself such an overly ambitious program that you can't follow it. You could become discouraged and stop Kegeling altogether.

After a month or two of regular practice, you should feel a marked increase in control over your urine stream.

How to Kegel There are different types of Kegel exercises. For best results, include each type in every session.

Before you start Kegeling, first practice stopping and starting the flow of urine until you become familiar with your PC muscle and gain some control over it.

- Pumps: Squeeze the PC muscle, hold for three seconds, then relax for three seconds. Repeat as many times as you can, working up to thirty three-second squeezes at a time.
- Pulses: Squeeze and relax the PC muscle quickly in a fluttering motion. Start slowly at first, aiming for regular contractions rather than speed. Over time, you'll be able to do this at a faster, even pace.
- Bear downs: This variation also tones your lower abs by adding a gentle bearing-down motion to your contractions-relaxations, as if you're having a bowel movement. Hold and release for three seconds at a time, working up to thirty sets. Don't be too forceful; the operative word is *gentle.*

A Sample Kegeling Session Exhale as you give a short squeeze. Squeeze the PC muscle and anal sphincter fifteen to twenty times at approximately one squeeze per second. Make sure that your buttocks muscles are not contracting too; it's important to isolate and work only the PC muscle and anal sphincter. Gradually build up to two sets of seventy-five one-second squeezes per day.

Squeeze the PC muscle and anal sphincter for a count of three. Relax for three counts. Work up to contracting for ten seconds, and relaxing for ten seconds. Start with two sets of twenty three-second squeezes each and build up to seventy-five ten-second squeezes.

When you become practiced and toned, add very gentle bear downs. After releasing the contraction, push down and out gently with your PC muscle and anal sphincter, as if you were having a bowel movement. Start with two sets of twenty bear downs, and build up to seventy-five bear downs.

You can work up to three hundred Kegel repetitions a day, combining short and long squeezes and bear downs.

After two months of 300 Kegel squeezes daily, you will have a strong, well-developed PC muscle. You can maintain that tone, flexiblity, and control by doing only 150 repetitions several times a week.

Easy Strengtheners and Stretches

Most fertility-boosting disciplines emphasize a pliant spine and flexible muscles—keys to eternal youth and increased fertility. A flexible lower spine is particularly essential because it enhances the function of the nervous and hormone systems. A rigid, tight spine and pelvis obstruct the flow of energy, blood, and other substances that should circulate freely through your reproductive organs. In other words, a body that's been sculpted to perfection at the gym may conform to popular notions of ideal male and female beauty, but it could be the barrier between you and a successful pregnancy. Unfortunately, many of us suffer from fertility-blocking rigidity.

The following simple movements drawn from traditional Taoist and yogic disciplines promote energy flow, strength, flexibility, and hormone balance. When you are performing these movements, always remember to inhale through your nose and exhale evenly through your nose. Never hold your breath and take your time.

Pelvic Tilt This exercise promotes strength, flexibility, and increased circulation in your lower abdomen.

Step 1: Lie on your back, bend your knees, and place your feet flat on the floor, hip-width apart.

Step 2: Squeeze your buttocks muscles at the same time you contract your abdominal muscles and press the small of your back into the floor.

Step 3: Still pressing the small of your back into the floor, exhale as you push your hips up toward the ceiling. Continue pushing your hips upward, maintaining the contraction in your buttocks and abs, while keeping your upper back and feet on the ground. Hold at the highest point for a moment.

Step 4: Slowly lower to the floor, unrolling your spine from the middle down to the bottom, and then lowering your buttocks.

Start out with five repetitions and gradually work your way up to twenty. Rest for thirty seconds, and then repeat.

Basic Body Stretch If you've ever seen a cat stretch, you know how wonderfully sensuous stretching can be. You can actually feel your body release tension; you automatically inhale more deeply, oxygenate your blood more thoroughly, release toxins, and promote healthy reproductive functioning.

If you add a nice loud sigh to your exhalations, you'll discover that the benefits are even greater: your body becomes even more relaxed, your capacity to stretch increases, and your mind feels more at ease.

Step 1: Lie on your back, arms comfortably extended over your head and a little out to the sides, legs extended and pointing slightly to each side.

Step 2: Push your heels forward, at the same time that you press your lower spine against the floor.

Step 3: Press and release your spine a few times to limber it up.

Step 4: Now that your lower spine has enjoyed a little stretch, press it against the floor again, at the same time stretching your arms away from your head and your legs in the opposite direction, extending your heels. Be sure to keep all four limbs on the floor. Inhale as you stretch, and feel your muscles release with each exhalation.

A terrific variation is to curve both arms and legs to the right side and then the left—making sure to keep the back pressed into the floor. This releases and stretches the sides of the torso, and gives the limbs an even greater stretch.

Sitting Forward Stretch This is another good stretch to keep your spine flexible and increase circulation in the pelvis.

Step 1: Sit comfortably on the floor, legs extended straight in front of you, a little less than hip-width apart.

Step 2: Use your hands to lift your buttocks off the floor and make sure that you're seated forward on your hips and that your spine is straight.

Step 3: Stretching from the hip joints rather than your back, lean forward, keeping the back straight. At the same time, extend your heels forward to maximize the stretch. Imagine you are bringing the lower abdomen closer to the thighs.

Don't worry about how far you bend. Hold and take ten slow, deep breaths. You should feel the stretch in the back of the calves and hamstrings.

Backbend Stretch This exercise stretches and loosens the muscles all along the front of your body, increasing circulation to the pelvis. Do not do this if you have chronic lower back problems.

Step 1: Sit on a mat or cushion placed on the floor, buttocks on heels, thighs together, knees bent, and lower legs tucked under your thighs.

Step 2: Place your hands behind your hips to support you.

Step 3: Squeezing your buttocks tightly and pushing your hips forward, slightly arch your upper body backward, stretching the front of your thighs and your entire trunk.

Step 4: Stretch your chin up and slightly back, but do not let your head drop back all the way as this can damage the neck vertebrae.

Step 5: Hold the stretch as you inhale and exhale, slowly and evenly, at least ten times, feeling your body let go with each long exhalation.

The Yoga Way to Enhanced Fertility

Yoga means the union of body and mind through breath. This venerable Eastern discipline developed in India three to five thousand years ago and has many features in common with

Taoist postures and other Asian disciplines. Yoga has influenced modern holistic Western exercise and bodywork systems more than any other Eastern system.

The hatha yoga style, the form with which Westerners are most familiar, focuses on energizing, toning, and making the body more flexible. It consists of physical postures and breathing exercises that enhance overall physical health. But that doesn't make their benefits to your fertility any less potent. In our clinic, we sometimes recommend a regular yoga practice as part of a patient's daily or weekly routine as an effective way to secure good health and increase libido and fertility, especially when the stress and grind of IVF cycles turn the joys of lovemaking into a tiresome chore.

The main difference between yoga and Western exercise is that yoga emphasizes inner, not just outer health. The breath is also used to promote a greater sense of well-being and self-awareness and to facilitate performing the various postures. Unlike Western exercises, which can exhaust you, yoga never causes you to lose energy. Instead, you gain vitality and a more balanced and even energy. Yoga improves endurance and flexibility and promotes a stronger, more flexible spine and joints that enhance virtually every body function, including reproduction. Yoga also calms the mind and spirit, making not just your body but also your mind more supple and relaxed—ready for a successful pregnancy.

Although yoga teachers recommend practicing yoga at least one hour, several times a week, there are simple yoga postures ("asanas") you can do almost anywhere, and in very little time.

If it's possible, yoga should be practiced in loose clothing and at least two hours after a meal. However, a few yoga stretches or breaths, practiced anywhere, are better than not doing them at all. Yoga is not a competitive sport but a wonderful gift you can give yourself. Do the yoga postures at your own pace, and never force your body into any position it's not ready for. While yoga classes are strongly recommended so that you can be monitored and corrected, these easy and simple postures can be done almost anywhere:

Basic Eastern Breath Most of us in the West are shallow breathers who use only one-seventh to one-third of our lung capacity, robbing ourselves not only of oxygen, but also of the life-force energy, qi, we need for good health and maximum fertility. Few of us breathe deeply enough to fully energize our pelvic areas, yet when we do fill the pelvic girdle with fresh oxygen and qi, we bring energy, warmth, and circulation to the reproductive organs and glands. Virtually all Asian disciplines begin with the breath because it carries into and out of the body the universal energy that animates us and connects us to the greater whole. The Basic Eastern Breath is common to all Eastern disciplines.

Breath control means control of your energy, and its benefits are limitless. It helps also to visualize your pelvis as a balloon that inflates with air on inhalation, then deflates on exhalation. This deep-breathing pattern will energize and strengthen all the organs and glands.

For most Eastern breathing exercises, breathe in and out through the nostrils only unless otherwise instructed.

Step 1: Lie on your back with your knees bent, feet about hip-width apart and planted on the floor. Make sure the small of your back is relaxed against the floor. You may want to place a rolled-up pillow or towel under your knees to help your abdomen and back relax completely.

Step 2: Place your right hand gently on your lower abdomen and your left hand on your chest. Inhale slowly, evenly, and deeply, so that the right hand rises. Your left hand should stay still. As you exhale, your right hand should lower.

Step 3: Close your eyes to help you tune into your breath and become aware of how it is filling and energizing your body.

Step 4: Take several long, slow, deep breaths, trying to expand your abdomen a little more with each inhalation. Never force or hold your breath.

Step 5: Now imagine that each inhalation is filling your entire torso. The top is your neck and the bottom is your perineum. The sides include the circumference of your rib cage, stomach, and back.

Step 6: Inhale, first filling the bottom, then the top, and finally the entire circumference. Feel your rib cage expand as you inhale. Feel your genital area expand with energy and a deliciously alive sensation. Allow the space between your shoulder blades to relax open.

Step 7: As you continue taking long inhalations and exhalations, allow your breath to travel into your legs and arms, filling your limbs with vital energy, all the way down to the tips of your fingers and toes.

This breath may feel awkward at first, but after you've practiced it regularly for a while, it will become easy, familiar, and automatic. Great times to practice are in the morning before you get out of bed and start your day, and at night, before you drop off to sleep. The Basic Eastern Breath is a wonderful way to shed tensions at the end of the day and it also eases insomnia.

Once you are comfortable with this breathing exercise while lying down, practice it in a sitting position, always making sure that the abdomen is moving out with each inhalation and in with each exhalation, and that the chest stays still. Use the breath when you're stuck in traffic, in line, or any time you find yourself in a boring or stressful situation.

This is the basic breath you can use in every yoga asana, as well as Taoist postures.

The Mountain Pose This basic posture tones and energizes the entire body and helps you feel grounded. If you lack a sense of being rooted or grounded on this earth, you may suffer from the sense of self that prevents you from relaxing and "letting go," which, in turn, can impair your fertility.

Step 1: Stand with bare feet (if possible) hip-width apart. Focus your awareness on the sensation of being planted on the floor.

Step 2: Lift and spread your toes, then try to bring them back to the floor one at a time, starting with the small toe and moving to the big toe. This will give you a wider foundation.

Step 3: Starting with your ankles, and focusing on your spine, lengthen your body from the feet up, all the while maintaining that strong connection to the floor through your feet. Reach up from your ankles to your knees, from your knees to your hip sockets, from your hips to your waist, from your waist to your shoulders. Drop your shoulders as you lengthen your neck, tilt your chin slightly in, and stretch the top of your head toward the ceiling.

Step 4: Relax your shoulders, letting them "melt" downward, away from your ears. Allow your arms to hang loosely, fingers relaxed and soft. Like a mountain, you are rooted in the earth and reaching for the sky.

Standing Forward Bend This posture helps shed stiffness, rigidity, and tension by gently stretching the entire back of your body, thus increasing limberness and circulation all along your spine and throughout your body and promoting balanced hormone production and circulation.

Step 1: Assume the mountain pose stance.

Step 2: Bend your elbows and place your hands on the creases between your thighs and hips.

Step 3: Bending slowly and steadily from the hip sockets while keeping a straight back, lower your torso. At the same time, slide your hands down the fronts of your legs. Bend as far forward as you can while maintaining a straight back.

Step 4: Hold the posture and keep performing the Basic Eastern Breath.

Step 5: Allow your back to relax and let your head and neck dangle freely. Make sure that your neck, shoulders, and arms are relaxed.

Step 6: Hold the pose, remembering to breathe, as long as you are comfortable.

Step 7: When you are ready, come out of the pose by bringing your torso back up slowly, back rounded, hands on your hip sockets, until you are back in the mountain pose.

The Butterfly All yoga poses help stretch, relax, and energize your inner and outer body tissues; promote efficient circulation; and help the nervous system maintain healthy hormonal functioning. The butterfly has a more direct benefit on your reproduction functioning because it opens and softens the hip joints and stretches and tones the inner thighs—all of which sends qi, blood, and essential nutrients to your reproductive organs and glands.

Step 1: Sit on the floor and bend your knees. Bring the soles of your feet together, allowing your knees to splay open to either side of your body.

Step 2: Take hold of your feet and draw them as close to you as possible, keeping your spine tall and shoulders relaxed.

Step 3: Hold this pose and practice the Basic Eastern Breath, sending energy to your inner thighs and pelvic joints, and letting the stretch gently increase with each long, even exhalation. If you feel any discomfort, sigh as you exhale to help release that discomfort.

Step 4: Hold this pose as long as possible, filling your pelvic bowl with purifying air and energy, and exhaling your inner thighs and hip joints farther into the stretch.

Relaxation Pose Always finish your period of "activity" with this wonderfully calming posture.

Step 1: Lie on your back on the floor, your feet about two feet apart, arms slightly away from your sides. If you feel any discomfort in your lower back, bend your knees and bring them together. Or roll up a pillow and place it under your knees so that your lower back relaxes into the floor and your abdomen softens.

Step 2: Close your eyes and begin the Basic Eastern Breath. Turn your attention to your breath and follow its rhythms. Don't try to change anything; simply observe it. Is it slowing down? Is it becoming shallower? Are the exhalations longer than the inhalations?

Step 3: If you drop off to sleep for a while, that's okay. You can even practice this exercise in bed at night to send you off to dreamland.

Whether or not you fall asleep, you will come out of this pose feeling refreshed and energized. For those of you who find a daytime nap disorienting, the relaxation pose is a great substitute, especially when you have little time.

If you take a yoga class, be sure to ask your instructor to show you these additional fertility-boosting postures: squatting posture, knee and thigh stretch, chest expander, stick posture, knee squeeze, legs up, pose of tranquillity, crocodile, star posture, spread leg stretch, child's pose, and pelvis stretch.

Tantric Yoga Exercises

The tantric yoga style includes many powerful exercises that were designed specifically to enhance sexual energy and fertility. Tantric yoga views physical love as an expression of the spiritual union between male and female. Since yoga in general is about the union of opposites—yin and yang, body and mind, and so on—tantric yoga aims to reconcile the male and female principles both within you and between you and your partner. Tantric yoga is mainly known for choreographing sexual experiences that leave both partners feeling deeply connected with their inner selves, each other, and the entire universe. Not many people are aware that these exercises also are powerful aids for protecting reproductive health and enhancing fertility by promoting strength, flexibility, circulation, and endocrine balance.

Tantric Pelvis Swings Step 1: Place your knees and palms on the floor, fingers facing forward and spread apart, thighs and arms at right angles to the floor. Your neck should extend straight from your spine, neither tipping upward nor hanging downward.

Step 2: As you inhale deeply and slowly into your belly, tip your head and buttocks up, arching your back. Your belly should expand as it fills with air, and your pelvic girdle is relaxed and open.

Step 3: Exhale slowly, at the same time tightening your buttocks and tipping your pelvis forward and under. Your back should be rounded. Feel your pelvis muscles contract and tighten.

Step 4: Repeat this action: rhythmically inhaling, swaying your back and opening your pelvis; then exhaling as you tighten your pelvis and buttocks muscles.

Your partner can serve as guide, touching your buttocks and stomach to guide the direction of the swings, and making sure that you are not moving any other body parts, especially your thighs and middle. Your guide can also remind you to synchronize your inhalations and exhalations to the pelvis swings.

Pelvic Swings: Advanced Standing Version Step 1: Stand with your legs about hip-width apart. Feel your feet planted on the floor, your body weight evenly distributed between the heels and balls of your feet.

Step 2: Lift your toes, spread them apart, then let them float down to the floor. Feel how the bottoms of your feet, including the toes, are supporting your weight.

Step 3: Let your knees be loose and slightly flexed. Rock slightly back and forth between the front of your feet and the heels. Settle into a strong, grounded stance.

Step 4: As you inhale air into your belly, let your pelvis swing easily backward from the "hinge" of the hips. Do not move your waist or legs, just your pelvis.

Step 5: As you exhale, tighten your abdominal muscles to

expel the air slowly and steadily, at the same time contracting your buttocks and pushing your pelvis into a forward tilt.

Step 6: Use your arms to help you. Allow them to dangle loosely at your sides, swinging backward with your pelvis as you inhale, then swinging forward with your pelvis as you exhale.

Step 7: If you feel tight and "locked," that is, if your pelvis is unable to make these movements easily, keep practicing, observing your movements and correcting them in front of a mirror. Do this exercise regularly and you will loosen up.

Step 8: Once you are able to synchronize your breathing with the pelvic rocking and arm swings, bring in your PC muscle. As you inhale, allow your genitals to "open" and fully relax, imagining they are filling with life-giving energy. As you exhale, contract or "lock" the PC muscle and anus to prevent the qi you have gathered from leaking out.

Again, your partner can help by gently touching your hips and directing the movement of your pelvis to ensure it moves independently, without help from other body parts. He also can guide synchronizing your breathing and pelvic locks (squeezes of the PC muscle) with your hip swings. For the most benefits, practice this exercise every day for five to ten minutes.

The Way of the Tao

Until late in the last century, esoteric Taoist exercises were a secret held only by a select few. Now everyone has access to these postures that strengthen and revitalize the reproductive organs and glands by literally increasing and concentrating their energy. Although Taoist exercises have not achieved the popularity of yoga here in the West, they share many features, and these secrets from ancient Taoist masters can be an effective fertility booster.

Like yoga, Taoist discipline is about the art of self-healing through cultivation of life-force energy. Special Taoist postures give the dedicated practitioner an astounding degree of control over her body, especially the ability to build sexual energy and then transform it into healing energy.

The main reason Taoist postures cultivate sexual energy is that all the body's energy currents (the acupuncture meridians) pass through the pelvic area. If the pelvic area is blocked or weak, valuable life energy is lost, and all your organs and glands suffer, along with your ability to reproduce.

Most of us experience an abundance of life-force energy only in our youth. We do not know how to preserve and channel energy, let alone restore and multiply it.

Stress, poor diet, alcohol, drugs, and smoking, which offer only fleeting satisfaction, can gradually wear us out and weaken our infertility.

This loss of vitality and health usually takes time, so it is most often seen in middle and old age, when pelvic and rectal muscles have weakened, sagged, and loosened, allowing vital qi to drain out of the body, and making the older person feeble, prone to disease and dysfunction, and even senile.

Many relatively young people today also suffer from loss of vital life-force energy. The way of the Tao is among the best remedies for overcoming infertility and other debilitating conditions.

Taoist "exercises" strengthen and revitalize the reproductive organs and glands by literally increasing and concentrating their energy. They also allow you to orgasm either one of two ways: (1) you can discharge through the normal, "outward," genital release; or (2) you can learn how to have an "inward"

Taoist orgasm that retains all that aroused sexual energy within your body instead of discharging it, so that energy can be used to nourish, energize, and balance your organs and glands.

After steady practice of the postures you will learn here, you'll be able to retain energy you build up and transform it into a healing force. You will know how to literally move that energy from the ovaries or testicles up your spine, where it can heal your nervous system along the way, including your brain. After the energy reaches your brain, you will be able to send it down the front of your body so it can heal the other organs and glands in its path. Finally, you will move to the navel area, where it will be stored. This energy "pumping and moving" is accomplished through a combination of breath control, visualization, and flexing of the perineum or "qi" muscles, which include the PC muscle, the root of the vaginal walls, and the anal sphincter.

Unless otherwise instructed, use the Basic Eastern Breath while performing all Taoist exercises.

Fire Belly This breathing exercise helps you build energy in the area from about one inch above the pubic bone to about an inch and a half below the navel—the power center for all our body functions and activities, including reproduction. Either stand, feet apart and knees slightly flexed, or sit on the edge of a chair, back straight (men's genitals should be hanging free).

Step 1: Rub the palms of your hands together briskly until they are hot.

Step 2: Make gentle circular motions on your lower abdomen with your left hand, covering the area from just below the navel to just above the pubic bone. Do this clockwise several times.

Step 3: Rub your palms together to heat them up again.

Step 4: Use your right hand to massage the same area several times, in a counterclockwise motion.

Step 5: Make as many circles as you wish, making sure that you rub an equal number of times in each direction.

The Kidney Stimulator The kidney stimulator strengthens the kidneys, adrenals, and the entire glandular system that controls fertility. Taoist healers claim it counters impotence and premature ejaculation and keeps the skin smooth and beautiful.

Step 1: Sit or lie down comfortably. Rub your palms together briskly until they are very warm.

Step 2: Place your palms on the small of your back as you tilt your upper body slightly forward.

Step 3: Feel and visualize the energy flowing from your hands into your kidneys and adrenals.

Step 4: Massage the small of your back by rubbing up and down and then in a circular motion.

Step 5: Make a loose fist and softly pummel the small of your back for a few seconds.

Step 6: Repeat the rubbing and pummeling three times.

The Deer This powerfully effective practice increases and balances endocrine gland secretions and boosts energy levels for women and men. For women, this practice tones vaginal muscles, providing many benefits to the uterus and ovaries, as well as the entire hormone system.

Women should also practice the deer after bathing and preferably in the nude. Regular practice of this exercise helps prevent and even cure a host of reproductive organ and hormone imbalance–related problems, including infertility. Women add a "vaginal lock" to their PC-anal contraction.

Step 1: Sit on the floor, a couch, or a bed and draw the heel of one foot up to your groin so that it presses against the opening of your vagina and your clitoris. If your heel won't reach, place a hard round object, such as a child's ball, against the area, until you feel a gentle, pleasurably stimulating pressure.

Step 2: Rub your palms together briskly to build up heat, then cover your breasts with your hands and feel the heat penetrate every cell.

Step 3: Now rub your breasts gently but firmly in an outward, circular motion. Move the right hand in a clockwise direction, the left in a counterclockwise direction. Taoists recommend doing this for a minimum of 36 circles and a maximum of 306 circles, but you can circle as many times as you wish, making sure to circle in each direction an equal number of times. This outward massage clears congestion, preventing and even curing lumps.

Step 4: Rub your hands together briskly again. Reverse direction, rubbing your breasts in an inward, circular motion (right, counterclockwise; left, clockwise) to stimulate them. Together with the pressure on your clitoris and groin, the breast massage builds a warm, pleasurable sensation that stimulates hormone production.

Step 5: Tighten your anal and vaginal muscles and hold the contraction as long as comfortable. Relax, and then repeat.

After weeks of regular practice, you should be able to hold the contraction for a longer period. When you gain more control, you will be able to do the anal-vaginal locks while rubbing your breasts.

The following Taoist exercise shows you how to take the energy you've gathered and move it up your spine, to your brain, and then down the front of your body, healing and revitalizing every organ and gland system in its path.

Taoist Energy Transformation This powerful practice brings together control over three elements you've learned from the previous practices: the breath, the PC muscle, and the power of your mind. In this exercise, you will build and gather concentrated life-force energy that is stored in the ovaries and/or testicles, and then draw it up your body, where it will deliver vitality and healing. It can take some time to master, but it is well worth the effort. Once you have mastered this practice, you'll be able to direct your energy with your mind only, and your body will respond immediately. Take all the time you need to learn this exercise—several days, weeks, or months—and don't skip any steps. As your abilities progress, you will be accomplishing wonders for your vitality and fertility. This practice is best done in the nude.

Step 1: Sit cross-legged and rub the palms of your hands together vigorously until they feel hot.

Step 2: Practice the deer until you feel aroused.

Step 3: When your arousal reaches a high level, inhale deeply through your nose. At the same time, contract all your muscles—clenching the fists, clawing the feet down, clenching the jaw, tightening the back of the neck, and pressing the tongue firmly against the roof of the mouth.

Step 4: Activate the anal-PC muscle lock.

Step 5: Repeat several times, always maintaining anal-PC muscle locks to secure the energy you've built up.

Step 6: Whenever you feel out of breath, exhale and sense the energy building in your reproductive organs.

Step 7: Inhale and hold your breath at the same time that you begin to rhythmically squeeze and relax the anal and PC muscles in a pumping action. As you pump, see your energy as a golden light concentrated in your genitals. After each pump, exhale and relax.

Step 8: Inhale once more as you contract the entire genital-anal region and pull the golden light from the reproductive organs down to the perineum.

Step 9: Inhale once again, and pull the golden light to the base of the spine.

Step 10: On your next inhale, move it to the middle of the back, then to the neck until, finally, it reaches the top of the head. If, at any point in this process, you feel the energy lowering, stop to rebuild your arousal level by pumping.

Step 11: Circle the energy in your brain several times, first clockwise, then counterclockwise.

Step 12: Touch the front of your tongue to the roof of your mouth and stop pumping. Feel the energy you have generated flow down the front of your body from the crown of the head, past your nose, mouth, throat, heart, chest, and then into the navel area, thereby making a complete circuit of energy.

Don't overdo it and, of course, don't allow yourself to become stressed out with these exercises. The many different exercises noted and described here are merely examples of what you can choose to do. There is no need to attempt to practice all of them, and they are not certainly intended to be practiced one after another, in a marathon style. Choose one or two that appeal to you and you can practice regularly to relax and enhance blood and energy flow that will bolster your spirits and your body.

MANUAL THERAPY AND FERTILITY

A study published in 2004, in the online journal *Medscape General Medicine*, suggests that a particular type of physical therapy increases fertility. This type of bodywork is called the Wurn Technique, and it combines massage and physical therapy for the abdomen and pelvis. Another study shows that two-thirds of women who underwent the Wurn Technique became pregnant after undergoing IVF. (The typical pregnancy rate for IVF alone is 41 percent.) These women had all been infertile for five or more years.

The technique was originally developed to treat musculoskeletal and post-surgical pain, and it also is believed to relieve inflammation that can throw off normal reproductive function. Most women receive between ten and twenty hours of treatment for a cost of between $4,000 and $5,000 total. However, the right touch may not be limited to this technique, and we are just beginning to recognize all the healing powers of various types of massage and bodywork.

It has been proposed that there is a direct relationship between the condition of the lower back muscles and reproductive health. From this theory, Dr. Mojzisova of the Czech Republic treated infertile women with a combination of soft tissue and osseous mobilization techniques, post-isometric relaxation, and a home exercise program. For otherwise infertile women ages twenty-two to thirty, this treatment program resulted in a successful conception rate of 34 percent versus only 8 percent in the control group. (The results were published in volume 23 of the *Journal of Orthopaedic Medicine* [2001].)

DO-IT-YOURSELF ACUPRESSURE

Acupressure, or the Japanese term *shiatsu*, is like acupuncture, except instead of using needles, finger pressure is applied to specific points, called acupoints, in order to unblock life-force energy. The result is stimulated circulation, relief from pain, and revitalization of your entire being. Since all traditional Eastern healing systems view the body as an integrated whole, virtually any blockage in the body will have an adverse effect on reproductive health and fertility. It may be more pleasurable to have someone work on you, but you can also do it yourself any time, at your convenience, and you won't pay a single cent.

How to Apply Self-Acupressure

Always use firm pressure to stimulate the body's natural curative abilities. It may hurt a bit—especially if you need treatment on a particular point. But this slight pain should feel "sweet," as the Japanese describe the healing sensation. You can use your thumb, finger, palm, the side of a hand, or your knuckles to apply the pressure. Some professional acupressure practitioners even use their feet and elbows. Use prolonged, steady pressure; three minutes per point is ideal on the following acupressure points:

Sea of Vitality: *Shen Shu* (Bladder, 23), *Zhi Shi* (Bladder, 52)

Location: Altogether, there are four points. They are located on the lower back. The first set of points is located two finger widths away from the spine on either side. The other set of points are located four finger widths away from the spine on either side, at waist level.

Benefits: Relieves lower backache, fatigue, reproductive problems, impotency, and premature ejaculation.

San Ying Jiao (Spleen, 6)—Probably the Most Important Fertility Acupoint

Location: Midway between the inside anklebone and the Achilles' tendon, on the back of the ankle of each foot.

Benefits: Relieves sexual tensions, semen leakage, menstrual irregularity, and fatigue.

Caution: Do not use this point after the third month of pregnancy.

Three Mile Point: _Zhu San Lí_ (Stomach, 36)

Location: Four finger widths below the kneecap, one finger width from the outside of the shinbone on each leg. If you are on the correct spot, a muscle should flex under your finger, as you move your foot up and down.

Benefits: Strengthens entire body, especially the muscles, and aids the reproductive system.

Gate Origin: _Guan Yuan_ (Ren, 4)

Location: This is a single point located four finger widths directly below the naval.

Benefits: Relieves impotency, reproductive problems, irregular vaginal discharge, irregular menstrual periods, and urinary incontinence.

Do not use acupressure if there's a chance that you are pregnant.

Regular use of the venerable Asian practices you've learned about in this chapter and working the acupressure points we've described will not take much time away from your busy schedule, and the time you do spend will be well worth it, in terms of boosting your fertility. You even can work acupressure points while you're talking on the telephone or watching television. Making these healthy activities part of your daily life not only enhances your fertility in ways you may not have believed possible, it also counters the stress and sense of helpless frustration that commonly afflict couples challenged by infertility.

In the following chapter, you may be surprised—even shocked—to discover how much stress and frustration can sabotage your chances of a successful pregnancy. The good news is that coping with stress is far easier than you may have imagined, and we'll show you how.

Chapter 11

Change Your Mind and Improve Your Fertility Prospects

This last chapter of the book is the most important. Science has shown that your mind has much to do with your fertility, and you can easily change your mind to enhance your fertility. Those stories you may have heard about couples conceiving while on a cruise or during another type of holiday tell us an important fact: relaxation enhances fertility. I make use of this fact in my holistic approach with my patients because I know that mental and emotional stress can exert tremendous negative influence on health and fertility. Of course, infertility itself, as well as the new forms of its medical treatment can be major causes of stress.

So, which comes first—stress or infertility? It's a hard question to answer, as stress and infertility can form a vicious cycle. What's important is that stress reveals itself in physical, psychological, and behavioral ways. Common signs of stress may include anxiety, depression, insomnia, headaches, back pain, shortness of breath, abdominal pain, and, of course, irregular menstrual cycles—a common symptom of fertility issues. Stress also can cause health- and fertility-wreaking behaviors such as eating problems and bad lifestyle habits such as smoking or drinking. An international study of thirty thousand people conducted in the late nineties found that women are more likely than men to feel high levels of stress, which can lead to depression and anxiety.

We know that if you are grappling with the challenges of infertility, "Just relax and you'll get pregnant" may be one of the most exasperating examples of "positive spin" you'll ever hear, and understandably so. First, there's stress caused by trying for at least a year to become pregnant. Other negative emotions such as guilt, jealousy, and self-deprecation can be associated with infertility. Then, there's stress from undergoing the numerous and sometimes invasive tests to rule out fertility obstacles in you and/or your partner. If you work with a conventional fertility specialist, you may find yourself locked into a rigid timetable that dictates virtually every phase of conception and beyond, including when you should have sex, when to take medications, when eggs must be removed from your ovaries, and so on. Then, you have to wait nervously a few weeks to see if all this effort paid off in the form of a pregnancy. No wonder so many women—and their partners—who are confronted with this situation find themselves more stressed out than ever before in their lives.

Yet there's truth in that old bromide, "Just relax and you'll get pregnant."

Before we tell you how to turn bad stress into good, let's explore "bad" stress a bit further. Bad stress is also known as *distress*. Modern "do it all" women are quite familiar with distress. In general, today's women suffer from distress caused by tremendous pressure to be perfect—as wives, employees, daughters, friends, and mothers. The stress of perfectionism sets us up for failure and a host of negative emotions, including anxiety. So even if you began the baby-making process in a relatively stress-free, optimistic state of mind, you have to find ways to overcome the tendency to isolate yourself socially, and to deal with the lowered self-esteem, and the disappointment and frustration from lovemaking that doesn't seem to lead to conception and birth of a child.

As we explained in the introduction to this book, your mind—rather than your body—may hold the key to your successful pregnancy. Modern medical science is learning more about the connections between psychology and physiology every day. For example, recent evidence suggests that the activation of brain regions associated with negative emotions appears to weaken immune response. Other studies show that the more stress a woman is under, the more likely she is to experience pain during her menstrual period, possibly because stress raises levels of progesterone, a hormone that counteracts the effects of estrogen. So the right solution is to reduce negative stress at the same time that you take steps to build your resilience to stress you cannot avoid.

Harvard researcher Alice Domar, along with Dr. Herbert Benson, from the Mind/Body Medical Institute at the New England Deaconess Hospital established that mind training can improve infertility as early as 1990. They reported in the December 1990 issue of *Fertility and Sterility* on fifty-four women who completed a behavioral treatment program for infertility. By eliciting the relaxation response alone, the researchers demonstrated significant decreases in anxiety, depression, and fatigue, as well as increases in vigor. Perhaps most important, 34 percent of these women became pregnant within six months of completing their program.

According to TCM, stress can impede free flow of energy, blood, and other fluids, thus setting you up for the imbalances that lead to infertility. Another way to explain the harmful effects of stress on reproduction is to refer back to that hormonal chain of command that controls virtually all body functions. Stress causes your brain to signal for the body to release stress hormones. If stress is chronic, the continual rise in levels of these stress hormones throws off the balanced and smooth functioning of the hormonal chain of command (specifically, the hypothalamic-pituitary-ovarian axis) that controls a normal menstrual cycle and fertility. As we tell the patients who come to our clinic, if you are looking for a cure for stress and anxiety, look no further than your own mind. With a little knowledge and practice of the strategies you will learn a little further along in this chapter, your mind can become your most powerful ally against stress and its negative effects on fertility.

STRESS, YOUR BRAIN, AND HORMONE BALANCE

Let's take a closer look at how stress can disrupt the delicate processes and balance maintained by the hormonal chain of command. Emotions are handled by your mind-body complex along the same route followed by the hormonal chain of command that controls menstruation and reproduction, starting with the limbic part of the brain. First, the limbic system recognizes an emotion—fear, for example. That message of fear is translated via the hypothalamus to the pituitary gland, and then on to the rest of the body. The body responds to this message with increased perspiration, heart and pulse rate, adrenal hormone production, and decreased digestive rate—all symptoms of what is commonly called the basic "fight or flight" response. Hormones secreted by various glands, as well as chemical messengers called neuropeptides, mediate all these body responses. So it's easy to understand how strong emotion can interfere with balanced hormone production by diverting your mind-body energy away from that job. This is how chronic states of fear, worry, anxiety, or anger can throw off hormonal balance and impair fertility.

For example, you might be subject to continual stress from chronic anger over your job to the point where signals from your limbic system to the hypothalamus and then the pituitary, and so on are thrown off, upsetting the production of the luteinizing hormone (LH) that helps you ovulate regularly.

Typical stressful experiences that threaten fertility because they can cause hormonal imbalance include moving and job change. So, your best option is to cultivate a backseat attitude that includes accepting the fact that you cannot will yourself to conception. Do your best and leave God the rest—that is the lesson of the *Zen and the Art of Archery* fable.

Yes, you should put all the right elements for success into place, but then you should relax, let go, and be ready to receive and conceive. Remember: the element of chance plays a major role in reproduction.

Rebecca was in her early thirties and married for two years. Strictly speaking, she probably didn't qualify as "infertile" because she and her husband hadn't tried to get pregnant for over a year, but she was becoming worried. This couple was very serious about starting their family sooner rather than later. Rebecca had consulted a fertility specialist, and her husband had seen a urologist. During their first appointment at our clinic, we went over the major activities we advise patients to avoid at the same time they are trying to get pregnant, including overexercising or attempting to diet. Rebecca wasn't engaging in any of those activities. However, when we discussed the need to avoid stress and told her we usually advise our patients to avoid the news for the time they are trying to conceive, Rebecca was in disbelief. "But I am a journalist," she exclaimed. "What are we talking about here?" Rebecca knew her business, so it didn't take long to explain that the media prefer to report the negative, sensational, and outrageous. The fact that the sun is shining today in Timbuktu or that New Yorkers are cheerfully going about their business on a lovely autumn day is not news. The news media seem to believe that newsworthy subjects include only constant negatives on topics such as terrorism, war, impending environmental disaster, the housing bubble, rising inflation, soaring unemployment, and the like. This presents a problem for people like Rebecca, who are being infused with this constant barrage of negativity: Why would her body (or her deepest unconscious self) want to bear a child in a world that is so terribly destructive and bleak? The solution is switch off the news; but Rebecca could not turn it off—she was a news journalist. The solution we proposed was to counterbalance all the negative input with positive visualizations and self-hypnosis. She also managed to switch from her beat in international news analysis to entertainment news and stopped her professional habit of engaging in late-night CNN reports for entertainment. While you cannot change what news the media churn out, you can voluntarily and consciously tune out the news that would otherwise seep into your subconscious and create an undercurrent of danger that hampers fertility. Just eight months after following our advice—and without any other therapy—Rebecca happily reported she had successfully conceived and delivered a baby boy.

The second step you can take to reduce stress is by making any necessary changes to manipulate what your mind perceives. As you know, you and your partner enjoy job security, you live in a comfortable home—disaster is not at your doorstep, but you can still be subject to the message of endless distress in our world. If you live in an overcrowded environment, that can signal to your unconscious that there are already too many of us, so you do not need to make any more. Newspaper headlines or the nightly television news reports on subjects that include crime, wars, unemployment rates, rising interest rates, the impending burst of the real estate market bubble, and global warming, as well as other imminent environmental calamities, including floods, famines, earthquakes, and tsunamis. The reports broadcast a negative message to your unconscious, telling it this is not a good time for you to reproduce.

Before the advent of modern communications—radio, movies, television, telephone, and the Internet—we were far less aware of what went on outside our immediate environment. We may have heard vague stories about events that happened somewhere else, but they didn't seem as real or as vivid as the nightly parade of the images and sounds of human cruelty and suffering we now experience at the flick of a TV remote power button. As you know, the problem is that our unconscious can't tell distance or time or distinguish between images from real life and the media. So, as we take in information from many thousands of miles away our unconscious may interpret this information to be present and immediate, and thus signals our bodies that our world is stressful and threatening, so do not reproduce. This can happen despite your conscious willingness or desire for a baby. What can you do to defuse this conflict between your unconscious and your conscious desire?

You, the individual—the woman or the man—may want to reproduce, but in order to do so, you must counter powerful unconscious forces that may tell your body to behave otherwise. What can you do?

How to Defuse Environmental Stressors from the Media

This chapter offers you many strategies for easing stress, but you can short-circuit one major source of stress with a simple action. Switch off anti-reproduction messages from the environment simply by turning off the flow of images of war, starvation, and other potential disasters to our society, our environment, and our race. Avoid the media, at least during the time you're trying to get pregnant. Instead, read comics and rent comedies or other diverting DVDs and tapes. In a sense, you have to fool yourself—at least that deepest part of your mind—by reducing the negative information you take in and absorb.

RELAXATION STRATEGIES

One of the best strategies you can adopt to help you through the fertility process and even maximize your chances of a successful pregnancy is to learn how to induce a relaxation response in your mind-body complex. It's far easier than you may believe.

No matter what technique you use, relaxation training frequently focuses on the breath and muscle relaxation, and then progresses to allowing thoughts to drift into and out of the mind, rather than hanging on to any worrisome thoughts that are already there. In this relaxed state, you can distance yourself from negative thoughts and emotions about your fertility and make room for the positive images of guided visualizations that replace all that anxiety and negative thinking.

The ideal mind state is "relaxed attention": you are alert and concentrated on what is happening inside you, but at the same time, you are uninvolved with what may be happening on the outside.

It is important to understand that this kind of relaxation means time alone in a quiet environment where you will not be disturbed, even by the telephone or doorbell. It does not mean lying on the sofa with your feet up, mesmerized by the television or radio.

During deep relaxation, refrain from any other activity.

Research has shown that for deep relaxation to be effective, you must have at least one period of relaxation daily lasting a minimum of fifteen to twenty minutes. After a month of regular practice, all you will have to do is give yourself a one-word cue, such as *relax*, and your body will immediately respond accordingly.

In a state of relaxation, thoughts occur less frequently and do not become fixations. Your breathing becomes slow and regular, and your muscles feel deeply relaxed. This state might be characterized by a heavy, weighty sense of your body, or the opposite—a light, floating sensation. People often report feeling quiet, focused, and passive. All these sensations are usually indications that you're deeply relaxed. There are many techniques to achieve relaxation. But remember that these are just tools and the goal is one. So, although we list a number of practical tools here for you, there is no need to use all of them; just choose or try one technique that you find useful. As long as you reach the goal of relaxation, whichever technique helps you get there is good enough.

Contraction-Release

One of the most common methods of relaxation is based on the principle of contraction-release in which you tense and then relax successive muscle groups of your body. When tensing a group of muscles, hold them as tightly as possible, then let go and relax completely. Best results are gained through regular practice. If you wish, record these instructions on a cassette tape, which adds an added self-help element because your own voice is helping you through the exercise. Also, listening to calming music while doing any of the relaxation exercises can be helpful.

- Arrange your body in a comfortable, receptive position. Lying on your back on the floor is preferable, but you may sit in a chair if you wish. Uncross your legs and extend your arms along your sides, palms facing up.
- Take three long, full inhalations, exhaling completely

each time. Feel your body let go of tension with each exhalation.

- Clench your right fist and hold the tension there, tighter and tighter. Study the tension in your right fist as you keep the rest of your body relaxed.
- Drop the tension and allow a sensation of relaxation to flow in. Observe the difference between relaxation and tension as a pleasant, heavy feeling floods your hand—into your palm, into each finger.
- Now, clench your left fist, then release the tension in the same manner as above.
- Clench both fists and straighten both arms, tensing the muscles. Hold the tension. Observe the tension. Now release the tension in both arms and let them drop to your sides. Observe the warm, heavy feeling of relaxation flowing into your arms, down your elbows, through your wrists, into your palms. Feel yourself letting go, relaxing. Take a long, deep breath. Exhale slowly, becoming even more relaxed.
- Take another long, deep breath, filling your lungs. Hold the air in your chest, observing the tension created. Now exhale slowly, observing the walls of your chest loosen as the air is pushed out. Continue relaxing and breathing freely and gently.
- Tighten your abdominal muscles by pushing them up and out as far as they can go. Hold the tension there and study it. Release the abdominal muscles and allow the feeling of relaxation to flow into each muscle. Continue breathing freely and easily. On each exhalation, notice the pleasant sensation of relaxation spreading throughout your body.
- Tense your buttocks and thighs by pressing down as

hard as you can and by clenching your buttocks muscles together. Hold the tension and study it. Release and allow a deep, soothing feeling of relaxation to flow in.

- Tense your lower legs by clawing both feet down as hard as you can and pinching your buttocks muscles together. Hold the tension and study it. Release and allow a deep, soothing feeling of relaxation to flow in. Breathe in and out easily and allow relaxation to flow throughout your body.
- Tense your back and shoulders by pinching your shoulders together and arching your back off the floor. Hold the tension and let go, allowing your back to drop gently back to the floor. Feel the relaxation spread.
- Roll your head back and forth very gently from side to side, releasing the muscles in the back of your head.
- Tense your facial muscles by sticking out your tongue as far as it will go, closing your eyes tightly, and wrinkling up your forehead. Hold the tension, then release, allowing warm relaxation to flow through your scalp, forehead, eyelids, cheeks, jaw, even your tongue.
- Now, allow your body to experience heaviness, as if it's boneless and only the floor is keeping you from sinking. You may, at this time, make a mental inventory of the parts of your body you have contracted and released, telling yourself as you go through your body that each part is heavy, warm, and relaxed.
- When you are ready to re-enter the waking state, begin by gentling wriggling your toes and fingers, gradually moving into whatever larger stretches your body wants.
- Roll to one side in a fetal position, place one palm on

the ground and push off, lifting your body comfortably and easily into a sitting position.

Ten-Minute Purifying Fire Visualization

This is an effective exercise in which your mind power and breath energize and cleanse your body of physical impurities, muscular tensions, and negative beliefs that impair your fertility. You can use the Basic Eastern Breath for all relaxation and visualization exercises. It also helps to create an audiocassette of the instructions, so you can play them back and relax to your own voice.

- Lie on your back, legs extended, about hip-width apart, arms slightly away from your sides.
- Focus your attention on the crown, or top, of your head.
- Now, shift your focus to the soles of your feet.
- Become aware of the space between the crown of your head and the soles of your feet. See that space as an empty container waiting to be filled and cleansed with the purifying energy of your breath.
- Inhale deeply through the bottoms of the feet as you visualize fresh, pure, sparkling life-force energy entering and moving up to fill the container of your body. With each inhalation, that life-force energy moves farther and farther up.
- As the purifying light-energy passes through your body, see all physical impurities and tensions, all fatigue, all negative beliefs and emotions, as dried autumn leaves. The life-force energy is gathering up these leaves and carrying them upward.

- As you exhale slowly and evenly, see the dried leaves—impurities, negative thoughts, and other obstacles—exit through your mouth and nostrils, then combust in a brilliant flame that incinerates them completely.
- Keep inhaling the leaves upward and exhaling them into a fiery nothingness until no more leaves are left, and you are full of sparkling light and energy.

Quick-Fix Stress Breaks

These quick fixes relax and focus your mind and release stress in anywhere from one to five minutes.

- Chant om. Om (pronounced "aaah-om") or another repetitive word (*peace* or *calm*) will quiet your mind.
- Breathe easy. Inhale and exhale through your nose, creating a rhythmic pattern that lengthens progressively. Inhale for four counts, exhale for four counts, then inhale for five counts, exhale for five counts, and so on. Do not hold your breath in between inhaling and exhaling.
- Move and repeat. Any repetitive movement—walking, swimming, tai chi, chi gong, or yoga will induce a meditative state.

Tantric Color Meditation

Tantric practitioners and increasing numbers of Westerners know that color can exert a powerful effect on our minds and bodies. Scientists have even shown that violet increases the activity of the female sex glands. So this exercise uses color to increase the energy and health of your body, especially the reproductive organs and glands. Again, recording and playing back the instructions in your own voice adds to the benefits.

- Sit in a comfortable cross-legged position or in a straight-back chair, making sure your spine is straight and shoulders relaxed.
- Close your eyes and visualize radiant colors—brilliant rays of red, orange, yellow, green, blue, indigo, and violet—pouring over you in a warm, life-giving flood. Feel each of these luminous energies penetrate every cell and tissue.
- Relax, letting your entire body go limp for a few moments.
- Sit upright again and exhale all the air from the lungs, forcing it out by contracting your abdomen.
- Inhale slowly, expanding your abdomen. Hold your breath for the count of seven as you visualize the color violet (men should substitute red). See rays of violet (or red) flowing over your lower abdomen and genital area, then see violet (or red) covering the back of your head.
- Repeat this process three times.

Tantric yogis advise practicing this color meditation in front of an open window or outdoors, in sunlight.

HOW TO DEAL WITH NEGATIVE THOUGHTS

If you are unable to visualize a particular feeling or image, explore that block to discover why you are protecting yourself from that particular experience. Explore any strong negative feelings associated with that block—fear, anger, anxiety, or irritation. Do not try to suppress them. Ask yourself why you are feeling that way. This is how you'll discover what may have been blocking your fertility all along.

Two common negating thoughts are "I don't deserve to have a child" and "I'm not capable of having and raising a child." Do they sound familiar?

Once you uncover your negative thoughts and beliefs, you will realize that you were already playing out a visualization without even knowing it: a negative scenario about your ability to conceive, bear, and raise a child that fed you an endless loop of self-defeating suggestions. Don't be afraid to let *that* movie play out in your mind a few more times, until you can see it clearly as the lie that it is.

Give yourself the same sound counsel you would give a friend:

- Challenge the validity of your negative thoughts and the feelings they create.
- Get professional help if necessary, so you can finally overcome these obstacles to your happiness and replace them with more positive beliefs that will create a more fulfilling reality.
- Remember, you cannot enjoy a new outlook on your fertility and parenthood without first cleansing the mind of worn-out, unfulfilling patterns.
- Your will and energy are the engine of your visualization, so be open to doing whatever it takes to making your positive scenario real without forcing the issue. Even if you don't entirely believe that a guided visualization can change your ability to conceive and bear a healthy child, *pretend* that it will. The power of pretend cannot be undervalued. Over time, pretend develops into a habit of positive thinking and shifts the

creations of your imagination into the realm of genuine possibility.

CREATING YOUR OWN DE-STRESS PROGRAM

Remember: When it comes to stress, hormones, and your fertility, the toxic "input" (for example, a scene depicting the viciousness of war we may see on the evening news) we receive from the environment through any of our five senses is passed on, then circulated through our bodies via the interlocking web of our psycho-neuro-endocrine system, where that input is translated into the message that this is perhaps not a good time to conceive.

In our practice, whether stress seems physical, mental, or emotional in origin, the result is obstructed energy and fluid flow that end up in imbalances that can cause infertility. This is why all TCM strategies—acupuncture, nutrition, herbs, physical activity, meditation, and relaxation—work on both the physical and mental levels, restoring balance wherever it is needed.

A connection to yourself and others can be as important as nutrition and physical activity to your health and fertility, yet in today's busy world we often overlook the importance of making the right connections. We spend more time at work and less time with family and friends. It's a good idea at this time when you are preparing to create life to slow down and discover what's really important to you. You can accomplish all this and promote a "Zen and the Art of Fertility" attitude by integrating into your regular routine all the strategies you've learned here, in addition to other simple practices:

- Get needled. Don't forget that one way in which acupuncture promotes fertility is by relieving stress and depression. From an Eastern perspective, depression and anxiety result from obstructions in the mind-body system's qi, the animating force that flows throughout the universe and every life form. Acupuncture restores the flow by stimulating nerves at the insertion points, thereby relieving emotional pain caused by stress.

- Be still. Taking a brief timeout—even during the most stressful day—works wonders for your state of mind and curbs tendencies to worry. Quick meditations quiet your thoughts and provide instant calm. The simple visualization meditations you've learned in this chapter provide grounding, encourage self-awareness, and help you develop the ability to "go with the flow"—that is, accept the fact that, ultimately, you do not control the outcome in this situation. Even taking a daily walk on a favorite route and focusing on your inhalations and exhalations will produce a calming effect and help you remember to avoid unnecessary stress by taking your time in everything you do.

- Move, breathe, and stretch. Take walks in clean air. Regular practice of yoga, tai chi, chi gong, or other disciplines promotes healthy circulation, hormone balance, and calm without excessive effort. Infertility and infertility treatments can be stressful, and yoga and other Asian practices also help you redevelop a positive view of your body—including the parts with which you may be frustrated—so your view of yourself can expand beyond "pregnant, not pregnant." The word *yoga* actually means union, so partner yoga (find classes in your area) can be a great way to strengthen your union with your partner, especially if you are both stressed out by the infertility treatment process. Remember: Avoid strenuous, "burn type" exercise that depletes your energy and fertility.

• Journal. Your journal can be a catchall dumping ground for the trials and tribulations of life and infertility. When you're in a crisis, writing—however briefly—can neutralize negative emotions associated with the event. A journal is a place where you can write away stress and guilt and catalog your worries. You can help restore your sense of perspective by then lighting some candles, playing soothing music, and making a catalog of your blessings. Keeping a journal is also a way to become a better problem solver and a more effective partner to the doctors who are working with the two of you to overcome infertility. You may discover new, improved coping mechanisms or rediscover strategies you may have used in the past in order to deal with your current fertility challenge. Use the following prompts to get going:

When was the last time I faced a difficult situation, and how did I deal with it?
When was the last time I experienced joy? What brought it about?
How can I bring joy into my life now?
Who is important to me and why?
What are the reasons I have to be grateful?

• Designate "worry" and "worry-free" zones. Help yourself maintain the bigger picture by designating a little corner of your home as your "worry corner." Allow yourself twenty minutes of worry a day *only* in that corner and in that corner alone. Take an inventory of the things in your life that make you anxious. Get it right by distinguishing between minor annoyances and dire situations, between things that can be changed and those that can't. Now, change what can be changed and accept what can't.

Designate an entire room for your "feel good" zone, where

you are not allowed to worry, pay bills, or perform any other stressful activity. Read, try new hobbies, laugh with friends or your partner, or simply lie back and enjoy yourself. Your time in the "feel good" zone is unlimited, of course, because every time you relax, you reduce your body's production of stress chemicals such as adrenaline and cortisol, thereby promoting better hormone balance.

• Go outside your head. Becoming involved in a project within your community also restores your perspective. Volunteering a few hours a week at a soup kitchen or at a home for seniors is a good way to take an emotional vacation from your fertility concerns.

• Find your inner artist. Listening to music, painting, dancing, and singing are proven ways in which the arts can relieve anxiety and depression. Make a joyful noise in the shower, even if it is off-key. Singing is a great way to express yourself, plus it's linked to lower heart rate, decreased blood pressure, and, yes, reduced stress. Actually, you don't have to sing yourself or create art. You can immerse yourself in the pleasure of art created by others. Studies prove that exposure to the arts is enough to positively affect the parts of the brain that handle emotional responses. And, remember, the brain handles emotions via the same route that it sends the hormones controlling menstrual cycles and fertility. Music is also thought by researchers to lower anxiety-related brain chemicals. Dancing promotes higher levels of serotonin, which is associated with high self-esteem.

• Laugh it off. Stress is not a joking matter. According to the American Psychological Association, its potentially harmful effects are responsibly for nearly 90 percent of all doctor visits. Laughter is a great way to stay mentally grounded and keep your perspective, and has been proven to boost the activity of your immune system's natural killer cells and other defenses against infections. It also appears to reduce the amount of hormones such as adrenaline and cortisol that your body produces during times of stress. Finally, laughing helps expand capillaries, increasing flow of blood and oxygen to your entire body, including your reproductive organs. People need fun in their lives, especially if they're being treated for infertility. Try to get in at least a few minutes of laughter every day, especially with your partner, even if it's about your infertility challenges.

• Get enough zzzz's. I know, you heard this enough times from your mother. But the fact remains, your body needs sleep to bolster its defenses against stress. You need between seven and nine hours every night, preferably in an entirely dark room.

• Take a break to put more play in your day. Make blocks within your schedule for free time, enough time to see a movie, find a scenic spot for a picnic, plant sweet-scented flowers in your backyard, go for a short walk after dinner to gaze at the stars, dance to music from high school, or do something else that's fun. Having regular meals at a healthy restaurant so you don't have to prepare and serve all meals yourself is a great stress buster.

• Rub out stress. Studies prove that massage not only reduces muscular tension that can impede healthy circulation to your reproductive organs, it also sends oxygen to your brain to improve mental energy. In addition, it reduces stress, including anxiety and depression, by helping promote optimal nervous system function.

• Tune out. You are trying to persuade that innate survival instinct buried deep within you that now is the right time for you to have a baby. So avoid books, the Internet, magazines, radio, and television for as long as it takes to restore calm and to find your center. These are all sources of outside information that can broadcast messages of strife and turmoil, suggesting to your deepest consciousness that you should not reproduce. Instead, consider spending more time with family and friends, listening to music, and writing in your journal. It's no accident when an infertile couple who gives up and decides to take a cruise or other type of vacation together "miraculously" conceives during that relaxing period.

- Reach out. Finally, remember every day to give your partner or another person a hug. If the two of you feel as if you are having "sex on demand" because you're tied to the strict timetables of fertility treatment, you can easily lose track of the *real* reason the two of you wanted to create a life together—love. Or just hold someone's hand. We all need to be touched to improve health and well-being.

- Seek professional help. Don't be bashful if your stress or anxiety is such that you feel you may benefit from a therapist or a group therapy session. Many IVF treatment centers now have resident psychotherapists to help their patients who are undergoing fertility treatments. Many techniques are used, and one does not have to go into years of psychoanalysis in order to reap the benefits of professional psychiatric help.

Use Hypnosis for Relaxation That Enhances Fertility

The mind-body connection clearly can have an enormously positive impact on your odds of becoming pregnant, especially in cases where there is no obvious cause for the problem. But when you enter the world of assisted reproductive techniques, the added stress of finances, timing, doctor visits, frequent blood drawing, and other tests can hamper all your efforts to relax. Perhaps you are already aware that you need to address this issue, but can't figure out what technique to choose out of the many different stress-reducing practices that are offered. One simple method you can try is self-hypnosis, a practice supported by a growing body of research confirming its effectiveness in treating a variety of disorders such as chronic pain, anxiety, depression, and even infertility. Most recently, a small study showed that the use of hypnosis could double the success rate of IVF treatments.

- Practice. Please take the health- and fertility-destroying properties of stress seriously and practice tension strategies regularly, but also naturally so that trying to maintain your practice doesn't itself become a source of stress.

"Fifty years ago, medical practitioners would say that women were hysterical and that's why they were infertile," says Alice Domar, Ph.D., director of the Mind/Body Center for Women's Health at Beth Israel Deaconess Medical Center, part of Harvard Medical School. "With the advent of good diagnostic procedures, doctors began to believe that fertility was all physiological. What these physicians are not taking into account may be psychological factors that can contribute to the physiological ones.

Would you tell a cancer patient, 'Just relax and you'll be cured?' Procreation is the strongest urge in the animal kingdom and these women are having their instincts to procreate blocked—of course it's going to cause a tremendous psychological reaction."

Final Thoughts: Empowerment and Letting Go

The gradual coming together of conventional and alternative approaches to health, healing, and fertility is creating a more holistic approach to reproductive health based on the belief that mental, emotional, and physical aspects of fertility are inextricably intertwined. With all this new knowledge, the idea of treating only one aspect of the problem—the physiological—no longer makes sense.

We've covered the subject of infertility from both the conventional and traditional Chinese medicine perspectives so you would have all the information you need to make the right fertility choices. Both modern Western medical science and alternative approaches such as TCM have opened doors to new and exciting fertility options, and you now have valuable tools for taking more control over your reproductive destiny.

Always keep in mind that your own situation and reproductive needs are unique, and whatever your chances are, they can be improved substantially by following some of our simple advice.

This book has helped you to become involved in your reproductive process in a constructive way by offering all the information you need about your fertility condition and available treatment options. Now, you are equipped to work in partnership with your doctors. You can avoid being overwhelmed by the enormous distress that makes your dilemma seem worse by knowing you are not alone and by studying your options, but not necessarily by trying to assume ultimate control.

Again, the best state of mind to cultivate whenever you are challenged by infertility is a "Zen" approach in which you put all the right elements in place to receive and then, hopefully, conceive.

References and Recommended Reading

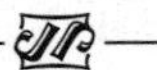

BOOKS

Appleton, Nancy. *Lick the Sugar Habit.* New York: Avery Penguin Putnam, 1996.

Atkins, Robert C. *Dr. Atkins' Health Revolution: How Complementary Medicine Can Extend Your Life.* New York: Bantam, 1990.

Bailey, Covert. *The New Fit or Fat.* New York: Houghton Mifflin, 1991.

Baker, Sidney MacDonald. *Detoxification and Healing: The Key to Optimal Health.* New Canaan, CT: Keats, 1997.

Balch, J., and P. Balch. *Prescription for Nutritional Healing.* New York: Avery Publishing Group, 2000.

Barnes, Broda. *Hypothyroidism: The Unsuspected Illness.* New York: Crowell Company, 1976.

Bechtel, Stefan. *The Practical Encyclopedia of Sex and Health: From Aphrodisiacs and Hormones to Potency, Stress, Vasectomy, and Yeast Infections.* Emmaus, PA: Rodale Press, 1993.

Benson, Herbert. *The Relaxation Response.* New York: Avon, 1990.

———. *Timeless Healing.* New York: Fireside, 1997.

Bland, Jeffrey. *The 20-Day Rejuvenation Diet Program.* New Canaan, CT: Keats, 1997.

Bratman, Steven. *The Alternative Medicine Sourcebook: A Sensible Guide to the Healers, Dreamers, and Liars.* Los Angeles, CA: Lowell House, 1997.

Brinker, Francis J. *Herb Contraindications and Drug Interactions: With Appendices Addressing Certain Conditions and Medicines.* Sandy, Oregon: Eclectic Medical Publications, 1998.

Brody, Jane. *Jane Brody's Guide to Personal Health.* New York: Avon, 1982.

Bruce, D. F., and S. S. Thatcher, M.D. *Making a Baby: Everything You Need to Know to Get Pregnant.* New York: Ballantine, 2000.

Bry, Adelaide, with Marjorie Bair. *Visualization: Directing the Movie of Your Mind.* New York: Barnes & Noble, 1972.

Canady, Ty. *What to Expect When You're Not Expecting: What You Need to Know but No One Told You.* iUniverse, 2003.

Carson, Rachel. *Silent Spring.* New York: Fawcett Crest, 1962.

Chan, Pedro. *Finger Acupressure.* New York: Ballantine, 1975.

Chang, S. *The Great Tao.* San Francisco, CA: Tao Publishing, 1987.

Charlesworth, L. *The Couple's Guide to In Vitro Fertilization: Everything You Need to Know to Maximize Your Chances of Success.* New York: Da Capo Press, 2004.

Chia, M., and M. Chia. *Healing Love Through the Tao: Cultivating Female Sexual Energy.* New Jersey: Healing Tao Books, 1986.

Childre, Doc Lew. *Freeze Frame.* Vista, CA: Planetary, 1996.

Colbin, Annmarie. *Food and Healing.* New York: Ballantine, 1986.

Collinge, William. *The American Holistic Health Association Complete Guide to Alternative Medicine.* New York: Warner Books, 1997.

Cousens, Gabriel. *Conscious Eating.* Patagonia, AZ: Essene Vision, 1992.

Csikszentmihalyi, Mihaly. *Flow: The Psychology of Optimal Experience.* New York: Harper & Row, 1990.

Dadd, D. L. *Home Safe Home.* Los Angeles, CA: Tarcher, 1997.

DeCava, Judith A. *The Real Truth About Vitamins and Antioxidants.* Brentwood, NJ: Brentwood Academic Press, 1996.

Domar, Alice. *Conquering Infertility: Dr. Alice Domar's Mind/Body Guide to Enhancing Fertility and Coping with Infertility.* New York: Penguin, 2004.

Dossey, Larry. *Healing Words.* New York: HarperCollins, 1993.

———. *Prayer Is Good Medicine.* New York: HarperCollins, 1996.

Douglas, A. *The Mother of All Conception Books: The Ultimate Guide to Conception, Birth, and Everything in Between.* New York: John Wiley & Sons, 2002.

Douglas, A., and J. R. Sussman. *The Unofficial Guide to Having a Baby.* New York: John Wiley & Sons, 2004.

Elias, Jason, and Shelagh Ryan Masline. *The A to Z Guide to Healing Herbal Remedies.* New York: Dell, 1995.

Ellison, Peter T. *On Fertile Ground: A Natural History of Human Reproduction.* Cambridge: Harvard University Press, 2001.

Epstein, Gerald. *Healing Visualizations: Creating Health Through Imagery.* New York: Bantam Books, 1989.

Feuerman, F. *Alternative Medicine Resource Guide.* Lanham, MD: Medical Library Association, 1997.

Fugh-Bergman, A. *Alternative Medicine—What Works: A Comprehensive, Easy-to-Read Review of the Scientific Evidence, Pro & Con.* Philadelphia, PA: Lippincott Williams & Wilkins, 1997.

Gach, Michael Reed. *Acupressure's Potent Points: A Guide to Self-Care for Common Ailments.* New York: Bantam, 1990.

Galland, Leo. *Power Healing: Use the New Integrated Medicine to Cure Yourself.* New York: Random House, 1997.

Gladstar, Rosemary. *Herbal Healing for Women.* New York: Fireside, 1994.

Golan, Ralph. *Optimal Wellness.* New York: Ballantine, 1995.

Goldberg, B. *Alternative Guide to Women's Health.* Puyallup, WA: Future Medicine Publishing Inc., 1993.

Goldberg, B., et al. *Alternative Medicine: The Definitive Guide.* Puyallup, WA: Future Medicine Publishing, Inc., 1993.

Goldfarb, Herbert A., M.D., with Judith Grief. *The No-Hysterectomy Option: Your Body—Your Choice.* New York: John Wiley & Sons, 1990.

Harvard Medical School. *Six Steps to Increased Fertility: An Integrated Medical and Mind/Body Program to Promote Conception.* Cambridge: Free Press, 2001.

Hay, Louise L. *Heal Your Body.* Carlsbad, CA: Hay House, 1994.

Indichova, J. *The Fertile Female: How the Power of Longing for a Child Can Save Your Life and Change the World.* New York: Adell Press, 2006.

———. *Inconceivable: Winning the Fertility Game.* New York: Adell Press, 1997.

Kabat-Zinn, Jon. *Full Catastrophe Living: Using the Wisdom of Your Body and Mind to Face Stress-Related Illness.* New York: Delta, 1990.

Keck, Robert. *Sacred Quest.* London, England: Chrysalis, 2000.

Kloss, Jethro. *Back to Eden.* Santa Barbara, CA: Woodbridge Press, 1983.

Kordel, Lelord. *Natural Folk Remedies.* New York: Putnam, 1974.

Lark, Susan M. *Fibroid Tumors & Endometriosis.* Los Altos, CA: Westchester Publishing Company, 1993.

Lee, John. *What Your Doctor May* Not *Tell You About Premenopause.* New York: Warner Books, 1999.

Levine, Barbara Hoberman. *Your Body Believes Every Word You Say.* Lower Lake, CA: Aslan, 1991.

Lewis, R. *The Infertility Cure: The Ancient Chinese Wellness Program for Getting Pregnant and Having Healthy Babies.* Boston, MA: Little, Brown, 2004.

Lowen, Alexander. *The Betrayal of the Body.* New York: Collier, 1967.

Lozoff, Bo. *It's a Meaningful Life.* New York: Viking Penguin, 2000.

Lyttleton, J., and S. Clavey. *Treatment of Infertility with Chinese Medicine.* New York: Churchill Livingstone, 2004.

Marti, J. E., and A. Hines. *The Alternative Health and Medicine Encyclopedia.* 2d ed. Detroit, MI: Gale Research, 1998.

McGuffin, M., C. Hubbs, and R. Upton. *American Herbal Products Association's Botanical Safety Handbook.* Boca Raton, FL: CRC Press, 1997.

Mendelsohn, Robert S. *Male Practice: How Doctors Manipulate Women.* Chicago, IL: Contemporary, 1981.

Micozzi, M. S., ed. *Fundamentals of Complementary and Alternative Medicine.* New York: Churchill Livingstone, 1996.

Mindell, Earl. *Earl Mindell's Vitamin Bible.* New York: Warner Books, 1979.

Monte, T. *The Complete Guide to Natural Healing.* New York: Bantam Books, 1994.

Moses, Marion. *Designer Poisons, How to Protect Your Health and Home from Toxic Pesticides.* Bethesda, MD: The Pesticide Education Center, 1995.

Murray, Michael T. *The Healing Power of Herbs: The Enlightened Person's Guide to the Wonders of Medicinal Plants.* Rocklin, CA: Prima, 1995.

Myss, Caroline. *Why People Don't Heal.* New York: Three Rivers Press, 1998.

Myss, Caroline, and C. Norman Shealy. *Anatomy of the Spirit.* New York: Random House, 1997.

Naparstek, B. *Health Journeys Guided Meditations: Help for Infertility.* New York: Image Paths, 2001.

Nissim, Rina. *Natural Healing in Gynecology.* London, UK: Pandora, 1986.

Northrup, C., M.D. *Women's Bodies, Women's Wisdom: Creating Physical and Emotional Health and Healing.* Rev. ed. New York: Bantam, 1998.

Ohashi, Wataru. *Do-It-Yourself Shiatsu.* New York: Dutton, 1976.

Oki, Mashahito. *Zen Yoga Therapy.* New York: Japan Books, 1979.

Oumano, Elena. *A Handbook of Natural Folk Remedies.* New York: Avon, 1997.

———. *Natural Sex.* New York: Dutton/Plume, 1999.

Parvati, Jeanne. *Herbs & Things: Jeanne Rose's Herbal.* New York: Workman, 1972.

Payne, N. B. *The Whole Person Fertility Program (SM): A Revolutionary Mind/Body Process to Help You Conceive.* New York: Three Rivers Press, 1998.

Pearl, Bill. *Getting Stronger.* New York: Random House, 1996.

Pelletier, Kenneth R. *Mind as Healer, Mind as Slayer: A Holistic Approach to Preventing Stress Disorder.* New York: Delta, 1977.

Pert, Candace. *Molecules of Emotion.* New York: Scribner, 1997.

Phillips, David A. *Guidebook to Nutritional Factors in Foods.* Santa Barbara, CA: Woodbridge Press, 1979.

Pizzorno, Joseph. *Total Wellness.* Los Angeles, CA: Prima, 1996.

Regenmorter, J. V., and S. V. Regenmorter. *When the Cradle Is Empty: Answering Tough Questions About Infertility.* Carol Stream, IL: Tyndale House Publishers, 2004.

Robbins, John. *Diet for a New America.* Tiburon, CA: H. J. Kramer, 1987.

———. *Reclaiming Our Health.* Tiburon, CA: H. J. Kramer, 1996.

Rosenthal, S. M. *The Fertility Sourcebook.* Cambridge, MA: Lowell House, 1995.

Salaman, Maureen, with James F. Scheer. *Foods That Heal.* Menlo Park, CA: Stratford, 1989.

Schmidt, Michael. *Smart Fats.* Berkeley, CA: Frog, 1997.

Scott, Julian, and Susan Scott. *Natural Medicine for Women.* New York: Gaia Books, 1991.

Selye, Hans. *Stress Without Distress.* New York: Signet, 1974.

Siegel, Bernie. *Love, Medicine, and Miracles.* New York: Harper-Perennial Library, 1990.

Skilling, Johanna. *Fibroids: The Complete Guide to Taking Charge of Your Physical, Emotional, and Spiritual Well-Being.* New York: Marlowe and Co., 2000.

Steinman, D., and S. S. Epstein. *The Safe Shopper's Bible: A Consumer's Guide to Nontoxic Household Products.* New York: Wiley, 1995.

Swire-Falker, E. *Infertility Survival Handbook.* New York: Riverhead, 2004.

Tierra, Michael. *The Way of Herbs.* New York: Washington Square Press, 1983.

Tyler, Varro E., and Steven Foster. *Tyler's Honest Herbal.* Binghamton, NY: The Haworth Press, 2000.

Warshowksy, A., M.D., and E. Oumano. *Healing Fibroids: A Doctor's Guide to a Natural Cure.* New York: Fireside Books, 2002.

Weed, Susun S. *The Wise Woman Herbal: Childbearing Years.* Woodstock, NY: Ash Tree, 1986.

Weiss, R. E. *The Everything Getting Pregnant Book: Professional Reassuring Advice to Help You Conceive.* Avon, MA: Adams, 2004.

Williams, C. D., M.D. *The Fastest Way to Get Pregnant Naturally.* New York: Hyperion, 2001.

Wisot, A. L., and D. R. Meldrum. *Conceptions and Misconceptions: The Informed Consumer's Guide Through In Vitro Fertilization and Assisted Reproduction Techniques.* Vancouver, BC: Hartley and Marks Publishers, 2004.

Yetiv, Jack Z. *Popular Nutritional Practices: Sense and Nonsense.* New York: Dell, 1988.

Zukav, Gary. *The Seat of the Soul.* New York: Fireside, 1990.

ARTICLES

Ceniceros, S, Brown, G. R. Acupuncture: a review of its history, theories, and indications. *South Med J.* 1998;91(12):1121–1125.

Chez, R. A., Jonas W. B. The challenge of complementary and alternative medicine. *Amer J Obstet Gyn.* 1997;177(5):1156–1161.

Eisenberg, D. M., et al. Trends in alternative medicine use in the United States, 1990–1997: results of a follow-up national survey. *JAMA.* 1998;280(18):1569–1575.

Miller, L. G. Herbal medicinals: selected clinical considerations focusing on known or potential drug-herb interactions. *Arch Intern Med.* 1998;158(20):2200–2211.

Torpy, J. M. Integrating alternative medicine into care. *JAMA.* 2002;287(3):306–7.

Ulett, G. A., Han, J., Han, S. Traditional and evidence-based acupuncture: history, mechanisms, and present status. *South Med J.* 1998;91(12):1115–1120.

MAGAZINES

Alternative Medicine Digest: (415) 435-1779
Natural Health: (800) 526-8440
New Age: (800) 782-7006
Yoga Journal: (800) 436-9642

Resources

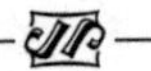

Alternative & Complementary Medicine Center (Health World Online):
www.healthy.net/clinic/therapy/index.html

Alternative and Complementary Medicine Links: (Emory University's MedWeb):
www.MedWeb.Emory.edu/MedWeb/FMPro

American Association of Acupuncture & Oriental Medicine:
(610) 266-1433

American Association of Clinical Endocrinologists (AACE):
(904) 353-7878; www.aace.com

American Board of Holistic Medicine:
(425) 741-2996

American College of Obstetricians and Gynecologists (ACOG):
(202) 863-2518; www.acog.org

American Foundation for Urologic Disease (AFUD):
(800) 242-2383; www.afud.org

American Holistic Medical Association (to locate a holistic physician in your area):
www.holisticmedicine.org

American Society for Reproductive Medicine:
(205) 978-5000; www.asrm.org

American Urological Association:
(410) 727-1100; www.auanet.org

Center for Alternative Medicine Research (Beth Israel Deaconess Medical Center, Harvard University Medical School):
www.bidmc.harvard.edu/medicine/camr/

Centers for Disease Control and Prevention:
(404) 639-3534; www.cdc.gov

Endometriosis Association:
(414) 355-2200; www.endometriosisassn.org

Health: Alternative Medicine Magazines:
www.yahoo.com/Health/Alternative_Medicine/Magazines/

The Health Resource (medical research reports):
(800) 949-0990; www.thehealthresource.com

MEDcetera (medical research reports on rare and chronic diseases):
(800) 497-0490

MedSearch (medical research reports):
(888) INFO-400; www.MedSearchInc.com

National Center for Complementary and Alternative Medicine (NCCAM):
at http://nccam.hih.gov/health

The National Infertility Association:
(617) 623-0744; www.resolve.org

National Institutes of Health:
(301) 496-4000; www.nih.gov

National Women's Health Information Center (NWHIC):
(800) 994-9662; www.4woman.gov

Natural Healthcare Hotline (for information on herbs and other supplements):
(303) 449-2265

Rosenthal Center for Complementary and Alternative Medicine (for resources on alternative medicine research, especially women's health):
www.rosenthal.hs.columbia.edu

Society for Women's Health Research:
(202) 223-8224; www.womens-health.org

www.webmd.com (general medical information)

SUPPLEMENTS AND HERBS

Abundant Life Herbal Supply: (510) 939-7857

A Catalogue of Herbal Delights: (800) 879-3337

AmeriHerb, Inc. (800) 267-6141

Emerson Ecologics: (800) 654-4432

Gaia Herbs: www.gaiaherbs.com

Phillips Nutritionals: (800) 582-8461

Phyto Pharmacia: (800) 553-2370

Vitamin Direct: (800) 468-4027

Vitamin Discount Connection: (888) 848-2110

The Vitamin Shoppe: (800) 223-1216

Vitamin Trader: (800) 334-9300

The Vitamin Zone: (800) 583-1187

ORGANIC FOOD AND NATURAL CLEANSERS

The Allergy Store: (800) 824-7163

Harmony Products: (800) 869-3446

Natural Lifestyle Supplies: (800) 752-2775

Natural Products: www.realgoods.com

Self Care: (800) 345-3371

Index

About the Authors

Raymond Chang, M.D. is an internationally respected physician-acupuncturist uniquely trained in traditional Chinese medicine as well as contemporary Western medicine. He is an acknowledged pioneer in the field of alternative and complementary therapy programs. He trained at Yale Waterbury and New York Cornell Hospital and attended at Memorial Sloan Kettering Cancer Center from 1987 to 1998. He currently attends at New York Presbyterian Hospital and is also the medical director of the Meridian Medical Group and president of the Institute of East West Medicine. Chang lectures frequently on the topics of alternative cancer, infertility, and herbal treatments.

Elena Oumano, Ph.D. is a Communications professor at City University of New York. She also has authored many health books, including *Natural Sex*, and is the co-author of *Healing Fibroids: A Doctor's Guide to a Natural Cure.*

About the Authors